T0192791

Telehealth Nursing

Dawna Martich, MSN, RN, received her bachelor's and master's degrees in nursing from the University of Pittsburgh and has been practicing as a nursing education specialist for adult learners for three decades. After working in neurology, postanesthesia recovery, home care, and physician practice management, she served as a direct telephonic nursing care provider for an organization with a satellite office in Pittsburgh, Pennsylvania.

Shortly thereafter, Ms. Martich became one of several training managers for a telephonic organization. Although the organization had a specific computerized clinical documentation system, it lacked approaches to help nurses transition from direct care to the telephonic care environment. After orienting hundreds of telephonic nurses in Pittsburgh, Arizona, Hawaii, Seattle, and Baltimore, it became clear that telephonic nursing care would stay as a viable avenue in the health care industry. She structured approaches to help nurses fine-tune their communication skills and develop an ease with computerized documentation.

Ms. Martich's other experience includes preparing student learning materials and ancillary materials for nursing publications and creating NCLEX-style practice questions for students preparing to sit for the state board of nursing examination. She has actively participated in creating content for online learning courses for RN–BSN, RN–MSN, and RN–DNP programs. She also served as the director of continuing nursing education for an online continuing education company, ensuring that learning material adhered to the American Nurses Credential Center criteria. Her most recent accomplishments include consulting to aid a start-up personal care agency with policies, procedures, quality improvement, human resources, and financial management functions. She can be reached via e-mail: dawna .martich@att.net.

Telehealth Nursing

Tools and Strategies for Optimal Patient Care

Dawna Martich, MSN, RN

SPRINGER PUBLISHING COMPANY

NEW YORK

Copyright © 2017 Springer Publishing Company, LLC

All rights reserved.

No part of this publication may be reproduced, stored in a retrieval system, or transmitted in any form or by any means, electronic, mechanical, photocopying, recording, or otherwise, without the prior permission of Springer Publishing Company, LLC, or authorization through payment of the appropriate fees to the Copyright Clearance Center, Inc., 222 Rosewood Drive, Danvers, MA 01923, 978-750-8400, fax 978-646-8600, info@copyright.com or on the Web at www.copyright.com.

Springer Publishing Company, LLC
11 West 42nd Street
New York, NY 10036
www.springerpub.com

Acquisitions Editor: Elizabeth Nieginski
Senior Production Editor: Kris Parrish
Composition: diacriTech

ISBN: 978-0-8261-3232-1
e-book ISBN: 978-0-8261-3233-8

16 17 18 19 20 / 5 4 3 2 1

The author and the publisher of this Work have made every effort to use sources believed to be reliable to provide information that is accurate and compatible with the standards generally accepted at the time of publication. Because medical science is continually advancing, our knowledge base continues to expand. Therefore, as new information becomes available, changes in procedures become necessary. We recommend that the reader always consult current research and specific institutional policies before performing any clinical procedure. The author and publisher shall not be liable for any special, consequential, or exemplary damages resulting, in whole or in part, from the readers' use of, or reliance on, the information contained in this book. The publisher has no responsibility for the persistence or accuracy of URLs for external or third-party Internet websites referred to in this publication and does not guarantee that any content on such websites is, or will remain, accurate or appropriate.

Library of Congress Cataloging-in-Publication Data

Names: Martich, Dawna, author.
Title: Telehealth nursing : tools and strategies for optimal patient care /
  Dawna Martich.
Description: New York, NY : Springer Publishing Company, LLC, [2017] |
  Includes bibliographical references and index.
Identifiers: LCCN 2016047388 | ISBN 9780826132321 | ISBN 9780826132338 (e-book)
Subjects: | MESH: Telemedicine | Nursing Care
Classification: LCC R855.3 | NLM WY 100.1 | DDC 610.285—dc23 LC record available at
https://lccn.loc.gov/2016047388

Special discounts on bulk quantities of our books are available to corporations, professional associations, pharmaceutical companies, health care organizations, and other qualifying groups. If you are interested in a custom book, including chapters from more than one of our titles, we can provide that service as well.

For details, please contact:
Special Sales Department, Springer Publishing Company, LLC
11 West 42nd Street, 15th Floor, New York, NY 10036-8002
Phone: 877-687-7476 or 212-431-4370; Fax: 212-941-7842
E-mail: sales@springerpub.com

Printed in the United States of America by Gasch Printing.

I dedicate this text to the following individuals:

- *My late parents, Daniel "Dragan" and Julia Martich—my first teachers, who taught me the value of hard work and patience, and gifted me with an understanding of the importance of lifelong learning. You are missed every day. I hope this text makes you proud.*
- *All patients and clients who are accepting of receiving telephonic nursing care.*
- *All organizations embracing telephonic nursing care.*
- *All current and future telephonic nursing care providers.*
- *All health care providers who question the validity of telephonic care. May this text change your mind. And if it doesn't, I tried my best to convince you.*

And last, but not least, I dedicate this text to my husband, Michael L. Egan. Without your patience, help, quiet strength, and love, none of this would have been written. Thank you for being my rock in the storm and voice of reality and reason. My heart is yours.

Contents

Preface   *ix*
Acknowledgments   *xiii*

Section I: Introduction   *1*

1. Evolution/History of Telenursing   *3*

2. Assessment Techniques: Communication and Active Listening   *13*

3. Professional Preparation for Telehealth Nursing   *39*

4. Patient/Client Perspective on Telehealth Nursing   *47*

Section II: Introduction to Body Systems   *67*

5. Integumentary System   *69*

6. Respiratory System   *89*

7. Cardiovascular System   *101*

8. Gastrointestinal System   *119*

9. Musculoskeletal System   *137*

10. Neurologic and Sensory Systems   *153*

11. Genitourinary System   *169*

Section III: Introduction to Body System Disorders   *183*

12. Disorders of the Integumentary System   *185*

13. Disorders of the Respiratory System   *193*

14. Disorders of the Cardiovascular System   *207*

15. Disorders of the Gastrointestinal System   *225*

16. Disorders of the Musculoskeletal System   *243*

17. Disorders of the Neurologic and Sensory Systems   *259*

18. Disorders of the Genitourinary System   *275*

19. The Patient/Client With Diabetes Mellitus   *289*

20. The Patient/Client With HIV/AIDS   *303*

Section IV: Additional Aspects of Telephonic Patient/Client Care   *311*

21. Patient/Client Care   *313*

22. Review of Laboratory Values and Diagnostic Tests   *331*

23. Documentation   *343*

24. Tools for Telephonic Care   *355*

25. Work Environments   *363*

26. Issues and Solutions   *371*

27. The Nurse as Client   *379*

Conclusion: The Rest of the Story   *389*
Index   *391*

Preface

Once upon a time, it was a dark and stormy night, the day before I was starting as a new telephonic nurse. I was scared to death and had no idea what I was supposed to do or how to do it. Over time, it became clear to me that telephonic patient/client care was and is an outstanding avenue to help many people.

Telephonic nursing care is not for everyone. For those nurses who want to stay in nursing but no longer want to provide direct care, this is not the text for you. Although you might not provide "hands on" care through this avenue, you will be providing direct care via ongoing assessment, follow-up, teaching, and support.

This text is divided into four sections. Section I sets the stage for providing telephonic care. First, you will read about the history of telemedicine and how telenursing was introduced into the field. Chapter 2 presents critical information on the techniques used to assess clients receiving telephonic care and includes an extensive review of communication and active listening techniques and the role of each in providing telephonic care. Section I ends with a chapter on what is needed to professionally prepare to become a telephonic care provider, followed by a chapter on the client's perspective on receiving care via this route.

Section II focuses on the individual body systems and how they can be assessed telephonically. After a brief anatomy and physiology review, questions used to assess the body system are provided. Approaches to use for special client situations are listed along with tips and techniques to enhance the assessment process. This section is divided into the major body systems: integumentary, respiratory, cardiovascular, gastrointestinal, musculoskeletal, neurological and sensory, and genitourinary. Although it is unlikely that you will need to assess every body system when assessing a telephonic client, these chapters will serve as a resource should the situation arise.

Section III focuses on illnesses, diseases, and disorders. The chapters in this section are also categorized according to the major body systems and can be used in sync with the chapters in Section II. Both Sections II and III feature algorithms to assess specific manifestations, along with practice exercises and case studies. You may note that "correct" answers for practice exercises and the case studies are not provided. This was done intentionally because there are a variety of answers and approaches that can be used to address the patient/ client situation. As you will read repeatedly throughout this text, there is more than one "right way" to do something, so there will be many "correct" answers to challenging situations.

Two specific disease processes are highlighted in Section II, with Chapter 19 focusing on the care of the client with diabetes and Chapter 20 focusing on the care of the client with HIV/AIDS. Diabetes was the "hallmark" disease selected for many start-up disease management companies in the 1990s and continues to be the focus for many of these companies today. Because it has been proven that this health problem can be successfully managed telephonically, devoting an entire chapter to the care and approaches was essential. Because several state telephonic care programs focus on the care of the client with HIV/AIDS, it was necessary to include a full chapter on this unique health problem.

Section IV provides "everything else" that a telephonic nurse might need to be successful in the role. The first chapter in this section focuses on patient/client care issues and teaching approaches. The next chapter reviews laboratory and diagnostic testing often prescribed for the client receiving telephonic care. An entire chapter is devoted to computerized documentation because this comes second only to the telephone when providing care using this approach.

The next chapter in Section IV focuses on the "tools" for providing telephonic care. Beyond the usual policy and procedure manuals, these include current nursing textbooks and lists of reliable websites, as well as other resources to support the nurse providing telephonic care in a variety of roles.

A chapter is devoted to the environments for providing telephonic care. Although there are only two—call center and home— each environment has particular challenges and advantages. These challenges and advantages flow directly into the next chapter, which addresses issues and solutions. As all nurses already know, there is no "perfect" work environment and not every patient is willing to accept telephonic care. This chapter provides strategies and techniques to help facilitate those particularly trying situations.

The final chapter of the text is devoted to you, the telephonic nurse. Through my years working with many outstanding nurses, I have seen and heard conversations in which nurses provided expert teaching and counseling to their clients but then neglected themselves.

Skipped lunches, missed breaks, and sitting for hours on end without stretching or walking all take a toll on the health of the telephonic nurse. This practice cannot become the expectation. Without you, the telephonic nurse, this aspect of the industry would not be successful. Read this last chapter carefully.

As this text was being created, I visualized myself in a training room environment facing a group of newly hired nurses. Each of these nurses had individual expectations for the position. Many wanted to "get out" of direct patient care. Others wanted to "try something new." And then there were others who just wanted to sit down for a while. As the weeks of training progressed, some of these new colleagues chose to leave. They did not realize what the position entailed, and they decided it was not going to fit into their career goals. Others "stuck it out" and became outstanding telephonic care providers. Many of these telephonic nurses have moved on to other health care provider roles in other organizations and continue to practice the highest quality of care.

Because a classroom full of nurses new to telephonic care was envisioned, a conversational approach was used. Every effort was taken to be as inclusive as possible; however, you might find that a situation important to you and in your telephonic work has been skimmed over or omitted. If so, please contact me so that it can be addressed in future editions of this text.

Keep in mind that reading this text from front to back might not be applicable to your situation. Allowing the reader to pick and choose the chapters according to his or her needs was a consideration as the content was being developed and designed. The most important thing is that you find this text helpful in providing quality telephonic care. If you find that it serves as a good resource, then the intention of the text has been achieved.

Best wishes to all who read this text, and may you always approach patient/client care with a sense of wonder and high expectation. Always remember that there is more than one right way to do something and tap into your higher creative powers when caring for your telephonic clients. You are an outstanding group of health care providers, all of whom I am proud to acknowledge as colleagues.

Dawna Martich

Acknowledgments

At first, I thought that this page would be blank, but the more I thought about it, it became clear that I have many people to acknowledge. These people may be completely unaware of their contribution to this text; however, I will be forever grateful for their guidance, direction, ongoing communication, and help.

I would like to first acknowledge the organization that provided me employment as a telephonic care nurse. I had no experience in the industry, but they took a chance on me. I know that they are still a successful company, and I continue to track their progress and wish them well.

The second acknowledgment is to the outstanding members of the leadership teams that have either directly or indirectly supported me in the various roles that I held while actively employed in the telephonic industry: Tom C., Bob S., Chris C., Debbie A., Pete K., Barbara G., Sheila H., and Katrina W.

Next I would like to acknowledge the various telephonic care colleagues who either held leadership positions, served with me in the classroom, were the front line in providing exceptional telephonic patient/client care, or held call center support positions: Cathy E. (the Red-haired nurse), Mary Ann L., Kim Z., Sandy H., Toni M., Joanna G., June Marie L., Carol Ann S., Carol M., Tammy H., Natalie S., Michele G., Cynthia B., the "ladies of July" including Martha A., "the groupies" including Trish S., Venus T., and the late Denise C., Patty G., Linda B., James S., Carol P., Tamara P., Madeline L., Dorothy M., Carla D. (who was in orientation with me on our first day), Lisa C. (HR), Kathy F., Bob P., Janice C., and Mimi W., (our dieticians), Clyde R., Bill W., Susan Y., Debbie Mc., Sally N., Luanne H., Janice P., Janie M., Linda L. W., Sandy S., Peggy V., Diane B., Ria R., Karen D. W., Rose, Alexis C., Ruth Ann De., Laura M. B., Susan C., Nikki Z., Connie P., Barbara S., Kimberlee M., Melanie P., Barrie Ann T., Karen H. R., Claudia S., Carol C. Z., Karen G. Z., Cindi De., Christine "Chrissy" E. H., Laurie B. B., Susan K., Norma S., Bob "Fab," Amy B., Susan V., Michelle S. Mc., Carol H., Jo Ann A., Vickie L., Cathy N. (aloha!), Michelle C. S. S., Mary K. H., Diane F., Jennifer J., Janet Di., Anita T., Lynne H., Bonna P., June B., Paula W., Louise G., Linda B.-P., Ramona S.,

Shirley E., Linda S., Pat B., Diane P., Carol C.-S., Kitty L., Cindy D., Mauri D.-G., Linda H., Valerie G., Lori W., Wanda M., Christine H., Judy B., the IT guys (Norb, Bob, and the late Ken), Jeff C., Bill R., Linda "Lynn" B., Linda Y., Janis P., Anne W., Dawna S., Andy P. (hanging out on the West coast), Cheryl G. (cotrainer in crime), the entire "BCBS Mass team," the entire "Oxford" team, and the entire "Cigna team." If I am omitting someone, please note that it is entirely accidental and poke me through Facebook or send me a tweet.

And last, but not least, I would like to acknowledge Elizabeth Nieginski and Rachel Landes for their gentle prodding, subtle guidance, cheerleading, and pep talks that I so desperately needed when my computer fried after a power surge.

Thank you, and many more years to you all!

Introduction

This text is not traditional in that it does not need to be read from front to back. It was created and designed to support nurses working in the telenursing industry. Although much more about telehealth and telenursing appears in later chapters, it is important to emphasize a few points here. First, working in telenursing is not for the nurse who "does not want to take care of patients anymore." This couldn't be further from the truth. Rather, in today's health care environment, with the need to do more with less and cut costs at every turn, telenursing represents an expansion of the industry, specifically, the specialty of nursing.

Further, this text was not created to support the "nurse on call" design of patient/client care. In true telenursing, patients are contacted on a routine basis. Plans of care are created. Assessments occur. Outcomes are measured. What differs is that the nurse and patient are not in the same room. In the "nurse on call" design, the patient phones into a call center with a particular problem or issue that is usually urgent or emergent in nature. In telenursing, the goal is to reduce or prevent urgent or emergent conditions by ongoing assessment, planning, teaching, and evaluation of outcomes.

Nurses employed in telenursing may have a set schedule for contacting patients. The frequency of the calls and subsequent care depend on the patient's health problems and learning needs. When providing care in this capacity, the nurse reinforces the medical plan of care, identifies and provides teaching to prevent disease and promote health, and strengthens the patient's ownership of health outcomes.

This text is not for every practicing nurse. It is ideally for those who are working within a telenursing setting and contacting patients enrolled in health plans, disease management programs, and wellness programs, which can include employees of various companies and health care systems. The beginning nursing student may find this text contradictory or confusing. This is because the techniques used when assessing and providing care via telenursing are altered. The traditional approaches used to assess, diagnose, plan, implement, and evaluate care do not always apply. This can cause conflict and confusion in a student or new nurse with limited hands-on clinical experience.

Most businesses using telenursing expect potential staff to have a predetermined amount of experience providing direct patient care. This is to ensure that the nurse can identify subtle nuances of disease manifestations and recognize when interventions are successful or need to be changed. The nurse with limited hands-on experience may feel lost or confused when the traditional approaches for problem solving and assessment are not available. Although this text will provide alternative assessment approaches, it would be beneficial if the nurse has had some experience providing direct patient care.

Even so, schools of nursing are becoming more creative at locating and establishing relationships for clinical experiences. As a practicing trainer in the telenursing industry, I established a clinical experience with a local university-based school of nursing for senior-level students. The students were assigned to mentor with nurses providing telenursing care. They "observed" the actions performed by the nurse, listened in on conversations and teaching sessions, participated in documentation, and actively identified teaching materials to support the patient's needs at the time of the call. The university considered this clinical practicum a success and desired to continue along the path for the years ahead.

As this text unfolds, keep in mind that the care of a patient through telenursing is an adventure. As with all adventures, the unexpected can occur. By knowing this in advance, the nurse in telenursing will have limited preconceptions and approach all patient care episodes as unique. Having basic knowledge of nursing science is integral; however, the interactions conducted with patients using this approach extend beyond the traditional therapeutic nurse–patient relationship.

Nurses who are hired in a telenursing role need a significant amount of training and continuing education. This text would be beneficial to use or provide as a guide during orientation of these employees. Each nurse would also benefit from having a copy of the text to use as a resource as patient care situations occur.

Keep in mind that telenursing is not for every nurse. Some nurses find the role challenging because of the desire or expectation to "do something" to help the patient. Nurses with this philosophy may find telenursing limiting their career development. Other nurses find telenursing the epitome of the nursing profession: opportunities to spend unlimited time talking, teaching, assessing, and partnering with patients as they journey to the goal of maximum wellness.

As you use this text, I ask that you keep an open mind and tap into your own powers of creativity. Remember that there is more than one "right" way to do something, and all nurses are capable of infinite creativity. Join me as we enter the world of telenursing.

CHAPTER 1

Evolution/History of Telenursing

LEARNING OUTCOMES

Upon completion of this chapter, the nurse will:

1. Realize that providing telephonic patient/client* care is not a new fad
2. Summarize the evolution of telemedicine and telenursing
3. Examine the basic nursing requirements to provide telephonic patient/client care

HISTORY OF TELEMEDICINE

Providing care to patients/clients through the use of communication equipment is not really new. It is only becoming more popular or used because of advancements in the telecommunication industry. It is thought that telemedicine was first used in the 1960s when the National Aeronautics and Space Administration (NASA) built health monitoring sensors into the astronauts' spacesuits to monitor the health effects of space travel.

Also in the 1960s, telemedicine was used within the psychiatric mental health care population, but in this case primarily for health care providers to communicate and consult with each other. The first documented use of telemedicine to provide direct patient care occurred in 1967 at Boston's Logan International Airport. A medical station was created, linking the airport with Massachusetts General Hospital, in order to provide care 24 hours a day.

During the decade that followed, NASA continued to play a role in telemedicine technology by employing satellites that transmitted information from Alaska (1971) or microwave technology to connect residents of an Arizona Indian Reservation with care providers (1972).

---

* The terms "patient" and "client" are used interchangeably throughout this text.

Also in the 1970s, the U.S. Department of Health, Education, and Welfare sponsored several hospital projects to demonstrate the use of telemedicine. The very next year two telemedicine programs were established: one in Boston for nursing home residents and another at Jackson Memorial Hospital in Miami, Florida.

Telemedicine continued to evolve over the next decades, focusing primarily on remote or rural areas that lacked consistent health care providers or facilities. During this time, telecommunication equipment advances were made to include adjunctive equipment or devices to aid in monitoring patient conditions. Examples of this equipment include home monitoring devices for blood pressure, weight, heart rate, oxygen saturation and blood glucose levels, and effectiveness of pacemaker functioning.

Personal computers have played a large role in the use of telemedicine today. Integrated cameras and applications encourage and support real-time interactions between health care providers and patients. The only challenge might be the patient's access to a device that can be used for these episodes of care.

IMPACT ON MEDICAL PRACTICE

Few people, if any, remember the days of physicians making "house calls." These visits were made by the neighborhood general practitioner to the homes of patients who were too ill to come to the office to be seen. As these visits fell away they were replaced by ambulance calls and trips to emergency departments.

Today, nearly every street block in major cities has an urgent care center. Community care centers are strategically planted to provide care to individuals who have limited access to financial resources or transportation. Pharmacies are incorporating "care centers" to enhance one-stop health care shopping—go to the pharmacy for an acute illness, receive a prescription, and shop while waiting for it to be filled. The need for "general practitioners" for everyday common ills has decreased.

With telemedicine, however, the philosophy of the "house call" is resurrected, but with a twist. Instead of having the physician physically arrive at the home, the patient/client and physician can connect through telecommunication equipment. The patient can be "seen" by the physician, who can conduct an assessment, make a decision about treatment, and direct the patient to either use a prescription or follow up with a "live" visit in the brick-and-mortar office setting. These "virtual" visits are enhanced for patients who have monitoring equipment attached to the telecommunication device, as the physician can evaluate additional data to support clinical diagnoses and decision making about treatment.

Even though this cutting-edge technology exists, telemedicine is not embraced by all in the medical field. Reasons for reluctance to use telemedicine include:

- The need to physically "touch" a patient prior to diagnosing an illness
- The need to use traditional tools; for example, stethoscopes, oto-scopes, ophthalmoscopes, and reflex hammers
- The fear of making a wrong diagnosis because of technological limitations
- The belief that medicine is not provided with a "cookbook" and should not be approached as such

But perhaps the greatest reluctance or fear of using technology to provide medical care is the impact it will have on the physician's income.

REIMBURSEMENT ISSUES

Once upon a time, physicians were paid for their services with cash. Then health insurance policies were created to pool financial resources. Over time, the cost of health care spiraled upward, and it became clear to the insurance industry that there just was not enough money to cover all of the costs of providing care.

In the 1980s, the insurance industry had the idea to designate a specific amount of money to pay for the care of a specific disease or diagnosis. Diagnostic-related groupings (DRGs) were born and regulated by the Centers for Medicare and Medicaid Services (CMS). To ensure that a patient's care did not exceed the amount of money that was allocated for a particular diagnosis or disease, health care organizations created tools and various care delivery systems to keep the patient's care "on track." Popular care terms during this time included primary nursing, case management, standardized care plans, and critical pathways.

But all patients do not fit into the confines of a set care map or standardized treatment plan. Patients needed longer hospitalizations and more frequent office visits. The amount of money that the average family physician received for patient care began a slow and steady decline.

Enter telemedicine. With this approach, the physician can be in one location and the patient/client in another. The patient does not have to travel to see a physician for a common ill or routine checkup for a known health problem. With this approach, the physician does not need to have large numbers of staff to collect data and maintain the office billing functions. However, the fear of losing even more income inched closer to reality.

Realizing the importance of telemedicine and the need to provide as much care as possible to the population within the United States, the CMS created guidelines for telemedicine reimbursement. Knowing that telemedicine care would be considered a covered benefit and payable through health insurance should help allay the physicians' fears, right?

AMERICAN TELEMEDICINE ASSOCIATION

In January 2013, the American Telemedicine Association published a document outlining Medicare reimbursement for telemedicine or telehealth services. Reimbursement would be provided for:

- Remote patient/client face-to-face services through live video conferencing
- Non–face-to-face services conducted through live video conferencing or store-and-forward telecommunication services
- Home telehealth services

Remote Face-to-Face Services

The CMS defines telehealth services to include those services that require a face-to-face meeting with the patient/client. Reimbursement is limited to the type of service, geographic location, organization delivering the service, and health care provider.

The service must be outside of a Medicare-defined statistical area; however, the health care provider can be located anywhere. Services that can be reimbursed include office visits, consultations, psychotherapy, and pharmacological management. The health care providers eligible to file for reimbursement include:

- Physician
- Nurse practitioner
- Physician assistant
- Nurse midwife
- Clinical nurse specialist
- Clinical psychologist

- Clinical social worker
- Registered dietitian or nutrition professional

And the originating sites under the Medicare rules are to be:

- Physician's office or practitioner
- Hospital
- Rural clinic
- Federally qualified health center
- Skilled nursing facility
- Hospital-based dialysis center
- Community mental health center

The amount of reimbursement to the health care provider is the same as that which would be paid for a "live" visit.

Non–Face-to-Face Services

These services, provided when the patient does not need to be present, include having a radiologist examine x-rays or a cardiologist study an electrocardiogram. The service is reimbursed at the same amount that would be paid if it was provided in a health care facility.

Home Telehealth Services

According to the CMS, home telehealth services are outside the scope of home care and are therefore not reimbursed. This does not mean that a home care agency cannot use telecommunication for patient care. Rather, it means the agency cannot bill Medicare/Medicaid for the service if provided through a televisit.

CURRENT REIMBURSEMENT FOR TELEMEDICINE SERVICES

Each year the CMS creates a list of services payable under the Medicare Physician Fee Schedule when provided through telecommunication. The most current services include:

- Psychiatric diagnostic evaluation with and without medical services
- Psychiatric visit with the patient and family; lengths range from 30 to 60 minutes

- Psychoanalysis with or without the patient and with or without the family
- End-stage renal disease visits with a patient receiving hemodialysis at a treatment center; various numbers of visits over 12 months to 2 years
- End-stage renal disease visits with the patient at home; various numbers of visits over 12 months to 2 years
- Neurobehavioral status examinations, initial and subsequent, with an individual patient, family, or a group
- Medical nutrition therapy with an individual or a group as an initial visit or subsequent visits
- Routine office visit with a new patient or an established patient
- Hospital care visit
- Nursing facility care visit
- Prolonged office or inpatient hospital visit
- Smoking cessation visit lasting at least 3 minutes up to greater than 10 minutes
- Transitional care visits 7 days after discharge and 14 days after discharge
- Diabetes management training individual and with a group
- Visits for a change in the diagnosis
- Alcohol treatment visits lasting between 15 and 30 minutes or longer than 30 minutes
- Inpatient follow-up care on days 15, 25, and 35
- Educational services for individual or group sessions
- Inpatient educational consultation 30, 50, and 70 minutes
- Counseling on tobacco use for 3 to 10 minutes or greater than 10 minutes
- Preoperative initial visit and subsequent visit
- Annual alcohol screening, 15 minutes
- Brief alcohol misuse counseling
- Annual depression screen
- High-intensity behavioral counseling, 30 minutes
- Intensive behavioral therapy for a cardiovascular diagnosis
- Behavior counseling for obesity, 15 minutes
- Telehealth inpatient pharmacy management

Currently, there are about 200 telemedicine networks, with 3,500 service sites in the United States.

Although physicians were slow to adopt telemedicine, its use is increasing.

INTRODUCTION OF TELENURSING INTO THE TELEHEALTH AND TELEMEDICINE FIELD

The first documented evidence of telenursing occurred in 1974 when Mary Quinn, RN, provided remote nursing care to patients who were at Logan Airport. Ms. Quinn was an employee of Boston Hospital's telemedicine center. Many consider this to be the date when the tele-nursing industry was born.

In the years since, little has been consistently studied or published about this up-and-coming niche within the nursing industry. In 2001, Charles C. Sharpe published the text *Telenursing: Nursing Practice in Cyberspace*, which focused on the legal, regulatory, and professional issues of the telenurse. As he points out, articles and studies on tele-nursing have been scant. The American Nurses Association published an official definition of telenursing in 1997 along with a set of professional guidelines for the nurse practicing in this type of setting; however, content to address the provision of patient care through this approach does not exist.

Sharpe claims that telenursing has been practiced in the United States for decades since the invention of the telephone and states that the industry truly started in the 1960s when nurses would talk to patients over the telephone. Although technically correct, telenursing is much more than contacting a patient as a courtesy call after hospital discharge or while recovering from surgery. Effective tele-nursing includes being able to adjust learned assessment and physical examination skills and apply these skills to an environment where the patient is not physically present. In the telenursing environment, care is provided through expert communication and listening skills.

Oftentimes, telenursing is grouped with telemedicine and tele-health even though each approaches health care through the use of tele-communications differently. Telenursing is much more than reminding a patient to see a health care provider for a follow-up appointment or helping a patient decide if an emergency department visit is required. To truly practice telenursing, the nurse must follow the nursing process when assessing, planning, implementing, and evaluating care.

An article by Laura A. Stokowski, published in 2008 and enti-tled *Healthcare Anywhere: The Pledge of Telehealth*, alludes to the intri-cacies involved when providing telephonic patient care. She explains that the practice of telenursing is unique and is similar to caring for a patient while blindfolded. Unfortunately, approaches to overcome the obvious barriers are not provided.

In 2000, the College of Registered Nurses in Nova Scotia published *Practice Guidelines for Telenursing*. Recently updated and released in 2014, this 14-page document provides a definition of telenursing, scope of practice and liability, confidentiality, and standards of care. Actual patient care approaches are limited to expert communication skills.

HEALTH CARE INDUSTRY CHANGES

The implementation of the Patient Protection and Affordable Care Act (ACA) of 2010 has revealed current and future deficits within the health care industry. One notable deficit is the number of providers needed to support the health care needs of insurance enrollees.

This legislation is providing increasing opportunities for nurses. Besides the obvious opportunities, such as the increased need for nurse practitioners and midwives, telenursing is being considered as an approach to meeting the needs for patient care. To help control the costs associated with office visits, physician practice groups are considering the use of telenursing to follow up with patient care needs. Overall, telehealth is contributing to the success of the ACA by providing another avenue to access care.

PREPARATION TO PROVIDE PATIENT CARE THROUGH TELENURSING

There is no one curriculum or learning tract within schools of nursing to "learn how to" provide telephonic patient care. Agencies or organizations hiring nurses for these roles identify specific criteria and characteristics for the position. An example of a position description for a telephonic nurse follows.

Position Description

- Provides care to individuals or defined patient populations through the use of telecommunication equipment in accordance with computer-based algorithms, protocols, or guidelines
- Uses critical thinking and communication skills to assess, plan, implement, educate, and evaluate patient outcomes
- Services are performed telephonically and interventions are documented in the computer application

Requirements

- Three years' experience as an RN
- Responsible and accountable for safe clinical practice, knowledge of customers, and regulatory expectations in the clinical area
- Permanent residence in a compact state
- Minimum of 3 years' clinical experience in acute care or medical office preferred
- Basic knowledge of nurse call center procedures
- Outstanding communication and telephone skills
- Basic computer skills/knowledge

Certifications/Licensure

- Licensed as an RN in good standing in the compact state of residence
- May be required to obtain licensure in up to 49 additional states

Additional Skills

- Comfortable communication using the telephone
- Demonstrates good customer service skills
- Good listening skills
- Demonstrates professional oral and written communications
- Demonstrates clinical judgment in accordance with the state Nurse Practice Acts
- Makes decisions that adhere to policy using basic critical thinking
- Self-motivated
- Acknowledges and accepts feedback on performance
- Asks for assistance and guidance as needed
- Adapts to change
- Demonstrates effective time management skills

KEY POINTS

- Logan International Airport in Boston, Massachusetts, is generally acknowledged to be the birthplace of both telemedicine and telenursing.
- NASA was the first organization that created and used telecommunication devices to monitor physiological functioning.

- Physicians are reluctant to implement telemedicine for fear of losing direct patient contact, making incorrect clinical decisions, and losing income.
- CMS defined and identified telehealth actions that would be reimbursed.
- Nurses do not "learn how to" provide telephonic patient care in basic nursing education.
- Telehealth, telemedicine, and telenursing all have important roles in today's health care environment.

BIBLIOGRAPHY

Allen, R. (2006). Electronic design. A brief history of telemedicine. *My TI Newsletter*. Retrieved from http://electronicdesign.com/components/brief-history-telemedicine

American Telemedicine Association. (2011). Telehealth nursing fact sheet. Retrieved from http://www.americantelemed.org/docs/default-document-library/fact_sheet_final.pdf?sfvrsn=2

American Telemedicine Association. (2013). Telemedicine and telehealth services. Retrieved from http://www.americantelemed.org/docs/default-source/policy/medicare-payment-of-telemedicine-and-telehealth-services.pdf?sfvrsn=14

Centers for Medicare & Medicaid Services. (2016). List of telehealth services. Retrieved from https://www.cms.gov/Medicare/Medicare-General-Information/Telehealth/Telehealth-Codes.html

College of Registered Nurses of Nova Scotia. (2014). Practice guidelines telenursing. Retrieved from http://crnns.ca/wp-content/uploads/2015/02/Telenursing2014.pdf

Kabir, J. (2014). Telehealth is the future. *Advance Healthcare Network for Nurses*. Retrieved from http://nursing.advanceweb.com/Continuing-Education/CE-Articles/Telehealth-Is-the-Future.aspx

Schlachta-Fairchild, L., Elfrink, V., & Deickman, A. (2008). Patient safety, telenursing, and telehealth. In R. G. Hughes (Ed.), *Patient safety and quality: An evidence-based handbook for nurses*. Rockville, MD: Agency for Healthcare Research and Quality.

Sharpe, C. C. (2001). *Telenursing: Nursing practice in cyberspace*. Westport, CT: Auburn House.

Stokowski, L. A. (2008). Healthcare anywhere: The pledge of telehealth. *Medscape Nurses*. Retrieved from http://www.medscape.com/viewarticle/581800

CHAPTER 2

Assessment Techniques: Communication and Active Listening

LEARNING OUTCOMES

Upon completion of this chapter, the nurse will:

1. Summarize the major senses used to provide patient/client care
2. Compare techniques used to provide traditional care with those used to provide telenursing care
3. Analyze the importance of effective communication when providing telephonic patient/client care
4. Examine the impact of distractions on active listening in telenursing
5. Demonstrate approaches to overcome communication and active listening challenges when communicating with a patient/client through telenursing

SENSES USED IN PATIENT/CLIENT CARE

The major senses are vision, hearing, touch, smell, and taste. Of these, the nurse providing traditional hands-on care uses sight, hearing, touch, and smell. These senses are well developed in nurses—finely tuned by constant assessment, reassessment, and evaluation of care.

Of these senses, the predominant one is sight. Nurses:

- Observe during a general survey
- Examine the skin
- Estimate wounds
- Analyze posture and gait
- Notice improvement or changes in physical status

The next most often used is touch. Nurses use touch to:

- Assess skin turgor and condition
- Pinpoint areas of pain
- Estimate muscle tone and atrophy
- Determine degree of edema

Imagine trying to console distressed patients without being able to touch them. You might question your effectiveness if you could not hug them good-bye as they left the hospital on discharge or hold their hand during a painful bedside procedure. Supporting the patient's psychosocial domain relies heavily on the sense of touch.

The next sense that is used extensively in patient care is hearing. Without this sense, nurses would not be able to:

- Auscultate lung and heart sounds
- Hear the anxiety in the patient's voice
- Analyze speech patterns associated with disease processes and conditions
- Respond to audible changes in breathing patterns and respiratory rates
- Answer patient questions

The sense of smell is used by nurses, but to a lesser extent in the provision of patient care. This sense is often used to reinforce information provided through other senses and helps the nurse to:

- Detect specific odors associated with disease processes, such as ammonia in liver disease and ketones in diabetic ketoacidosis
- Discern an infection within a wound

Taste is seldom, if ever, used in nursing care.

REVIEW OF TRADITIONAL ASSESSMENT TECHNIQUES

Early in our education, nurses learn the four techniques of assessment:

- Inspection
- Palpation
- Percussion
- Auscultation

These techniques capitalize on the use of the senses. For inspection, the nurse relies on the sense of sight. Smell is used to a certain extent during inspection and provides additional clues and indicators about health status, ability to provide self-care, and ability to maintain a safe home environment. Touch is used when assessing the skin, muscle tone, and other related general body structures. Without touch, the nurse would not be able to adequately inspect.

Touch is the primary sense used in palpation. Here, the hands are placed on various body areas to identify organ structures and boundaries. Palpation is also used to validate or support data collected through inspection. Without palpation, it would be impossible to:

- Assess pulses
- Determine the presence and size of masses
- Estimate the depth of edema
- Evaluate joint function
- Discern soft tissue swelling

Although percussion uses the hands to elicit a tone from a body area, the sense of hearing is predominant when using this technique. If hearing were absent, repeatedly striking over a body part would provide no useable information for the nurse. Of the assessment techniques used by nurses, percussion is most likely the one least applied. This is because it is instructed to be used primarily when assessing the lungs. Although instructed on the value of percussion when assessing other major body organs, the average nurse usually does not rely on percussion when assessing other thoracic and abdominal structures.

The final technique, auscultation, is often augmented with a stethoscope. Nurses auscultate for:

- Heart sounds
- Lung sounds
- Bowel sounds
- Vessel integrity

The purpose in reviewing the traditional assessment techniques has not been to encourage or reinforce their use in patient/client care. Rather, it is to emphasize how important the use of the senses is when determining patient care needs and to set the stage for how these assessment techniques will need to be altered when working in telenursing.

SENSES USED IN TELENURSING

Telenursing is unique in that the traditional approaches to assessment—inspection, palpation, percussion, and auscultation—need to be altered or cannot be used. Take a few minutes now and perform this exercise:

> Envision yourself sitting at home when the phone rings. The person on the line identifies herself as being with a health insurance plan or other care delivery system provider. She has your name, address, age, gender, and information about your health plan or employer. She begins talking to you and starts asking questions that expect you to divulge personal health information. Do you trust this person? How can you trust this person? Why is she talking to you? What health problem do I have that my doctor didn't tell me about? Should I answer this person's questions? Is this a scam or an attempt to steal my identity?

How comfortable were you when reading through that exercise? Would you talk to someone over the telephone about your health and care needs without seeing the person or understanding why the call was taking place? Would you be tempted to hang up and contact your health plan to find out what's going on or report the call to some authority?

As you might have concluded, the sense of sight is not an integral part of telenursing. You will not be able to "see" the patient to:

- Read nonverbal communication cues
- Examine the skin
- Determine the color of skin tone
- Observe for diaphoresis
- Visually inspect the ankles for edema
- Notice nail clubbing or the presence of a barrel chest
- Identify a spinal deformity, which could negatively impact respiratory excursion or gastrointestinal functioning
- Identify basic body shape that might indicate a potential risk for the development of metabolic syndrome or type 2 diabetes mellitus
- Analyze gait and stability with walking
- Discern patterns of bruising that might indicate a specific disease process from those obtained from a fall or episode of abuse
- Estimate the ease or challenges to complete instrumental or traditional activities of daily living
- Recognize sensory deficits through the use of a hearing aid or reading glasses

As you can see, the list of areas in which the sense of sight is used when assessing can go on and on. The sense of touch, however, is also absent in telenursing. Without this sense, you will not be able to:

- Feel skin temperature
- Palpate edematous areas
- Determine the point of maximum impulse when conducting a cardiac assessment
- Estimate organ borders
- Discern fremitus
- Palpate subcutaneous emphysema
- Reach for the patient's hand during times of stress

Before you run from the room screaming or slam the book closed, take a deep breath. Telenursing does not use rudimentary nursing assessment skills and techniques. Your skills will not be "lost" over time. You will learn new skills and techniques to replace those that rely on the primary senses of sight and touch. And you will learn to engage the patient/client to assist you during the assessment process.

FOCUS ON THE SENSE OF HEARING

In telenursing, the sense of hearing is predominant. Overall, you will be conducting patient interviews over the telephone and listening for patient responses. Of course, it is more involved than this statement, but to state the process in simple terms, in telenursing the mechanism of patient care is provided through talking and listening. Outstanding communication skills are essential.

Communication Approaches

When approaching a patient/client in a face-to-face setting, the nurse needs to keep in mind:

- Facial expressions
- Physical body language
- Tone and tempo of speech

In telenursing, the nurse needs to be aware of:

- Words/language used
- Tone and tempo of speech

Obviously, facial expressions and physical body language will not be involved in telenursing; however, keep in mind that these areas add to the quality of communication. When they are absent or not used, communication may falter or totally fail. To overcome the absence of these areas, the nurse needs to focus solely on the quality of verbal communication.

As a review, communication begins with a sender delivering a message to a receiver who, in turn, accepts the message and makes a response provided in the form of feedback. Effective communication needs a sender, a message, and a "willing" receiver. When starting out in telenursing, a willing receiver might be the most challenging part.

From the brief exercise explained earlier, how many people willingly answer the telephone and talk to someone they don't know about personal health information? How many television commercials have been created that warn older adults about potential telephone scams? How willing would you be to spend time with someone you don't know talking about the intimacies of your health problems and concerns?

In telenursing, the sender, or the nurse, has to be prepared to overcome these challenges. The nurse must use a tone that is pleasant and welcoming. Words must flow conversationally and not sound like someone reading a "script." The purpose of the call must be explained immediately before the patient hangs up thinking you are a telemarketer or someone trying to scam you into providing personal information to steal your identity.

Immediately upon the call being answered, the nurse needs to:

- Ask to speak to the patient
- Validate that the person on the phone is indeed the patient
- Provide nurse's full name
- Identify the company that the nurse is representing
- Explain the purpose of the call

The patient will undoubtedly have questions:

- How did you get my name and telephone number?
- Who are you again?
- Who are you with?
- Why are you calling me?

Yes, you did just provide all of this information when beginning the call; however, the patient was not hearing everything. Expect to repeat your opening statements over and over again. Remember, patients have no idea who you are. They will be concerned that their telephone number and personal health information is "floating" out there and will express caution and concern. You need to calm patients down and not feed into their anxieties. This means talking slowly, succinctly, and professionally. This is no time to inject humor or make light of the situation.

Answering the patient's questions accurately and calmly is the best approach to secure his or her tentative trust at this time. Be sure to:

- Repeat your name
- State the organization you are with or representing
- Explain the purpose of your call

Once you receive validation that the patient will continue with the call, you can then proceed to the purpose, which will most likely fall into the following categories:

- Health plan enrolled the patient into a health management program for a health problem identified during a recent hospitalization
- Employer enrolled the patient into a wellness program as part of a health care benefit paid for by the employer
- Health plan enrolled the patient into a health promotion/disease prevention program as an approach to reduce the cost of care based on bills received and paid

Now depending on the category of enrollment, the call may go in a variety of directions. The first step is to:

- Validate the patient's address
- Confirm best telephone number to use for future calls
- Confirm best day/time to connect with the patient

This might cause the patient to have additional questions or concerns such as:

- Am I sick and no one told me?
- How many calls are you going to be making to me?
- Why are you going to call me so much?

The responses to these questions will "depend." It depends on the type of program enrollment, the presence of a chronic illness, health issues identified after assessment, or frequency of using health resources for ongoing illness or wellness care. And the direction of future calls will be based on the results of a thorough assessment. Areas of assessment will be provided later in this text.

The Importance of Active Listening

Active listening is a skill in which the sender concentrates on the feedback or response provided by the recipient or receiver of the message. It involves consciously paying attention to every word said, the way the words are phrased, and the emotion or inflection added to the response.

Oftentimes, active listening takes a back seat during communication because the sender or receiver may be formulating a response while the other person continues talking. When this occurs, valuable information is not heard and may be lost. Depending on the direction of the communication, either the sender or receiver may become frustrated when this occurs because it appears that the other person is not "listening to" what is being said. Most of us have also experienced some version of the following scenario, in which someone is not participating in active listening because he or she is engaged in another task:

> You are talking while standing next to a person who is typing or inputting data into a computer. The person continues to type and repeats "uh huh" while you continue to talk. The person is not paying any attention—or is giving limited attention—to what is being said (the message) by you (the sender). After you leave the area the person continues to type and may or may not even recall what you said or whether it was essential, important, or a life-or-death situation.
>
> Suppose you do not leave the area, but instead wait for a response. Because the person typing was not paying attention, the response may be vague, scattered, or incorrect. You would likely then become frustrated at having to repeat everything that was previously said. Additionally, the person is now expected to focus on what you are saying; however, there is a chance that his or her thoughts are on anything but what you have to say. The person might be thinking about a response without hearing the complete message or trying to remember what additional information needs to be input into the

computer once the conversation ends. Either way, the message has been lost or distorted beyond the original intent.

Obviously, this is not the ideal approach to use when conducting a conversation with a patient over the telephone. All attention must be placed on the words being spoken by the patient. If necessary, it would be appropriate to jot down a few notes just to be sure that important areas mentioned are not lost. At no time, however, should the nurse focus on formulating a response while the patient is still talking.

Without a doubt, active listening takes energy and complete concentration. If the mind wanders and something important is missed, the patient will know or ask about it later. Not keeping track of the conversation and issues is one way for the fragile trust relationship to crumble within seconds.

EXERCISES TO IMPROVE COMMUNICATION AND ACTIVE LISTENING

Some nurses may think that exercising communication skills is a routine part of care or too basic to warrant attention. However, a brief review and practice is always beneficial. These exercises are best performed with two people participating.

EXERCISE 1

Arrange two chairs back to back so that it is not possible for either person to see the other. In this position, one person will play the role of a nurse and the other, the client. Use the following script for this exercise:

Nurse	Patient/Client
(Telephone is ringing and picked up.)	
	Hello?
Hello. Can I speak to Margaret Brown?	

(*continued*)

(*continued*)

Nurse	Patient/Client
	Who's calling?
My name is Denise. Can I speak to Margaret Brown please?	
	What is this about?
I cannot say unless I know that I am speaking to Margaret Brown.	
	Okay, this is Margaret Brown. Who are you and what do you want?
My name is Denise Jordan. I am a nurse with your health plan. They have identified you as a person who would benefit from participating in a health promotion program.	
	What? My health plan identified me as someone who would benefit from what? I'm not sick!
This has nothing to do with you being sick. A health promotion program is one that works with the patient to take active steps to prevent the development of a health problem in the future.	
	So what's this going to cost or how much more are my monthly premiums going to go up because of this?
This is part of your health plan. The cost for this is already included in your monthly premium.	
	So this is just something else that I am paying for that I don't want or need? Who do I have to call to get this taken off of my health benefit?

(*continued*)

(continued)

Nurse	Patient/Client
I'm not sure if that can be done. Your health plan has identified you as someone who is healthy. You don't use your benefits and as an added bonus, you have access to nurses to answer your questions and make sure that you are taking advantage of all of the steps available to keep you as healthy as possible.	
	So this isn't because I'm sick? This is because I'm well? Well that's different.
This is a program to keep you on the right track to ongoing wellness.	
(The nurse's manager walks by and places a piece of paper on the desk that says "come to my office as soon as you are done with this call.")	
	So what do I have to do now?
This is a program that makes sure you stay on the path to complete and lasting wellness.	
	You already said that. What do I have to do?
Well, first of all we need to validate all of your demographic information.	
	What's that? I'm not giving you my social security number. No way. If you say you're from the health plan then you already have that information!
No, demographic information is just to validate your address, telephone number, and the best day and time to call you going forward.	

(continued)

(*continued*)

Nurse	Patient/Client
(Several nurses are walking past the desk, signaling to the nurse to wrap up the call and hurry up because there's a mandatory meeting in the manager's office right now.)	
	Ok, well what do you have as my address and phone number and I will tell you if it's right or not.
Let's see, since I'm calling on Friday at 11 a.m. would this be a good time for calls in the future?	
	I guess but I thought you were going to start with my address and telephone number.
Right. I have your address as 1102 Agnes Lane, New Haven, Connecticut.	
	That's correct.
And your telephone number is XXX-XXX-XXXX.	
	That's right for now but my area code is going to be changing in 2 weeks.
Well, I thank you for your time and I will call again next Friday at 11 a.m.	
	Wait so that's all you're going to do right now?
(Dial tone.)	

After completing this script, consider these questions:

- What is the impact of minor distractions on a conversation?
- What could be done to reduce the impact of the message provided by the manager?

- What could be done to lessen the impact of the staff signaling that the call should be ended?
- How do you think the patient will respond the next time the nurse calls?

EXERCISE 2

For this exercise, use the same arrangement of the chairs. The roles of the nurse and client can be switched or changed with another staff member. The script for this exercise is as follows:

Nurse	Patient/Client
(Telephone ringing.)	
	Hello?
Hello. My name is Barbara. I am a nurse with Quantum Health, an organization that provides health promotion and education to recently hospitalized patients.	
	How did you get my name? I'm on the Do-Not-Call list in my state.
This is not a telemarketing, political, or charitable organization call.	
	Then what do you want?
Like I said, my organization receives the names of individuals who were recently hospitalized.	
	I wasn't in the hospital!
Was anyone else at this telephone number recently in the hospital?	
	I'm not answering that. Who do you want to talk to?
I'm calling to speak with David Hunter.	

(continued)

(*continued*)

Nurse	Patient/Client
	Which one? My husband is Sr. and our son is Jr.
The one who was recently hospitalized.	
	That would be my husband. Hang on.
(Background conversation: I don't know. Some nurse who wants to talk to you about you just getting out of the hospital.)	
	Hello.
Yes, hello. Is this David Hunter?	
	Yes, that's me.
My name is Barbara and I'm a nurse with Quantum Health, an organization that follows up with patients who were recently hospitalized.	
	How did you get my name and telephone number?
When you were hospitalized, you signed a general consent form agreeing to have follow-up conversations by a third-party organization.	
	When did I sign that? I don't remember signing that? (Side conversation with female voice: Did I sign some paper saying people can call me when I get home?)
Mr. Hunter. The consent was a part of a general consent form you most likely signed in the emergency department or at the admissions desk.	
	Well, I signed a lot of papers. Honestly I was so sick I don't remember everything that happened or what I signed.

(*continued*)

(*continued*)

Nurse	Patient/Client
That's understandable. Quantum Healthcare is an organization that follows-up with recently hospitalized patients to answer any questions during recovery at home and help you continue to get better from the recent illness.	
	I already know what to do. I got a mess of papers from the nurse when I was leaving yesterday and I have a doctor's appointment in 2 days. What help can you be to me over the telephone?
Our goal is simple: To keep you on the road to recovery and prevent the health problem from causing any more hospitalizations in the future.	
	I wonder how you're going to do that.
Through a series of telephone calls, we talk with you about your symptoms, your medications, your diet and exercise, and any follow-up tests or appointments scheduled by your health care provider.	
	And that's supposed to keep me out of the hospital?
Well, it's a matter of helping you manage your own health and health issues going forward. Our telephone calls will provide you with the tools to help keep you well.	
	That's fine but I can't talk long right now. The plumber just arrived.
So Mr. Hunter, is this a good day and time to call you next week?	
	Ah, yeah, that's fine. Okay. Bye.
(Dial tone.)	

After completing this exercise, consider the following:

- What distractors were in the patient's environment that influenced responses by the receiver?
- Why did the nurse elaborate about the Do-Not-Call list?
- What could the nurse have done to improve the patient's willingness to participate in future phone calls?
- What would be mandatory for the nurse to complete on the next call?

EXERCISE 3

For this exercise, keep the same physical arrangement of the chairs. The participants can switch or have different participants work with other groups.

Nurse	Patient/Client
(Telephone ringing.)	
	Hello!
Hello! My name is Arthur Greene. I'm a nurse with Maxi-Well, a health care organization that works with employees to improve or maintain their health. Is Gloria McKnight available?	
	I'm Gloria!
Well, Ms. McKnight, as I said, I am a nurse with Maxi-Well, which is an organization that telephones employees to discuss their health care needs, actions to take to improve their health, and provide guidance on health prevention activities.	

(*continued*)

(continued)

Nurse	Patient/Client
	This is so wonderful! You know, our HR person was telling us about this new benefit and I think it's terrific. Just the other day I was talking with my friend at work—she has so many health problems—and even though I don't, we both think this would be great. So do you have any diets or anything there that I can use that can help me lose some weight? I'm about 20 pounds overweight and my doctor is not happy with me. If I go back to see her in 3 months and I haven't lost any weight she is going to be so mad at me.
Before we get into that Ms. McKnight . . .	
	Call me Gloria.
Okay. Before we get into that, Gloria, would it be okay if I do a bit of housekeeping and get the standard questions out of the way?	
	Sure.
Can you validate your date of birth please?	
	February 3, 1951, but don't tell anyone! Everyone tells me that I don't look my age! I think it's because I eat right and exercise but I just can't lose any weight!
So are you located at 7 Vanadium Drive, Apt. 202, in Bridgeville, Illinois?	
	Yes, that's my address. Hey, are you going to be calling Doris next? She lives in my building too, a few floors up.

(continued)

(*continued*)

Nurse	Patient/Client
I'm not sure who else will be contacted. Is this a good telephone number to use for future calls?	
	Yes, and I can give you my cell phone number too, but I might not be able to answer it if I'm at work.
What day and time would be best to call you when you can be able to talk?	
	Mondays at 5 p.m. are the best for me.
Great. I'll write that down, Gloria. Thank you. So, to get started, we have a series of questions that serve as a guide to identify areas in which you might benefit to either maintain or improve your current health status.	
	Well, I know that I need to lose weight and you know Doris, she says that I don't exercise enough but who has time, you know? I do take my dog out for a walk every evening . . . do you have any pets? Well I walk about two or three blocks and then get home because I don't want to miss my shows. I just love my new cable company! There are so many great shows on and I make sure I see as many of them as I can.
Oh my, Gloria. Well let's focus on the areas that are available to you from your employer. The first area you mentioned already is weight management.	

(*continued*)

(continued)

Nurse	Patient/Client
	That's right. What kind of diets do you have available? I've tried all the major ones and I don't want to buy someone else's food. You know that stuff is all chemicals and tastes so bad. Doris is following something that she started a few weeks ago and she lost 5 pounds in 3 days, but then she hasn't lost any more so I don't want to follow that one . . .
There are no specific diets that your employer or our company advocates. We really just need to start with talking about your daily eating.	
	Hey, unless you give me a diet there's no way I'm going to be able to do this. Oh, wait a minute [sound of knocking], someone's at the door.
	(Muffled conversation heard at the door.)
	I have to go. My landlord's here to fix the heat.
Okay. Well, I'll phone again on Monday at 5 p.m.	
	Yeah, right. Okay.
(Dial tone.)	

After completing this exercise consider the following:

- What actions can be taken to keep the patient/client on track with the conversation?
- How might the conversation be changed to support the needs that the patient identifies as being the most important?

These are just three examples of types of conversations that can occur when providing telenursing care. Additional information about these situations and strategies to facilitate or overcome them will be provided later in the text.

CHALLENGING TELENURSING SITUATIONS WITH COMMUNICATION

A variety of communication patterns can occur during a telephonic patient/client care call. A few of the most frequently encountered situations are described here.

Patient/Client Hangs Up

Upon the call connecting, the nurse provides identification, name of the organization, and purpose of the call. The patient either immediately hangs up, says "I'm not interested," or something along the lines of "leave me alone."

The nurse should not continue to contact the patient. This information should be provided to the contracted organization for further investigation. Some organizations will follow up with printed and mailed material to patients who will not or who desire to not be contacted through the telephone.

Patient/Client Will Not Validate Personal Information

At the beginning of the call, the nurse needs to validate the patient's identity. Reasons for a patient refusing to validate identity include: fear of identity theft, unaware of being enrolled in the program, and not understanding the purpose of the program.

In these situations, the nurse should make every attempt to validate the patient's identification through the use of date of birth, address, telephone number, and if applicable, name of the health plan, employer, or posthospitalization disease management group. If still unsuccessful, the nurse should end the call and provide the name of the patient to the contracted organization for follow-up.

Patient/Client Wants Someone Else to Talk With the Nurse

At times, a patient may want someone else in the household to take the nurse's phone calls. Reasons for this occurring include: patient is older and does not understand the program; patient's health status is such that extensive talking on the telephone would be tiring; English is the patient's second language and medical terminology and nursing care is not completely understood; patient is a member of a couple in which one member has been responsible for health care (e.g., wife schedules appointments, follow-ups, and ensures medication compliance, for the husband or vice versa); and the patient is not of legal age to talk directly about health care needs (this would include all infants, children, and adolescents up until the age of 18 who are not identified as emancipated minors).

Before agreeing to talk with a family member regarding the patient's health status and care, the nurse needs the patient's permission. This can be verbal as long as it is documented in the patient's telenursing record. For patients with English as a second language, find out if the contracting organization has a relationship with a medical interpreter service. If so, and if the patient's primary language is represented, offer the use of interpreter services. For the patient whose spouse has assumed responsibility for health care, efforts should be undertaken to encourage the patient to take a more active role in self-health care practices and maintenance. Realizing that this might not occur, obtaining permission to talk with the spouse will be accepted. It is an expectation that for children and nonemancipated minors, the legal guardian or parent will be the person to communicate with during all calls. Efforts should be taken to validate the parent's/legal guardian's identity before divulging or questioning about personal health information.

CHALLENGING TELENURSING SITUATIONS WITH ACTIVE LISTENING

The issues with active listening in telenursing have much to do with the individual environments. The nurse might be located in a call center containing dozens of nurses all talking to clients at the same time. The patient most likely is at home and exposed to a variety of distractions such as the television, other people, children, pets, in the process of cooking, or helping other family members with projects or chores. Actually, the list of distractions in the patient's home can be endless. The next section reviews some suggestions to help with active listening issues

Noisy Telenursing Environment

Actions to help reduce the impact of a noisy environment during a call include:

- Increasing the volume on the telephone headset
- Facing into a wall or at a computer screen
- Closing the eyes while talking

Noisy Patient/Client Environment

Approaches to help facilitate active listening when the patient is distracted by a noisy environment can be borrowed from those found to be helpful when providing home care and include:

- Ask if the patient could turn down the television or preferably turn it off for the duration of the call
- Ask if other individuals in the patient's environment could talk softer or preferably ask if the patient can take the call privately in another room
- Ask if a barking dog can be let out of doors or if not able, ask if the call can be made at another time when the dog is least likely to be barking
- For crying babies or children, ask if someone is available to tend to the child's needs; if not able then offer the patient time to console the child or reschedule the call for later in the day or week
- If someone knocks at the patient's door or rings the doorbell offer the patient time to respond
- If the patient was expecting a call; however, a visitor, repairman, other intrusion occurs before or during the call offer to call back later or reschedule the call for another day and time

Active listening can also be affected by the patient's health status. If the patient seems distant or disinterested, the following is recommended:

- Ask if there is something on the patient's mind that is preventing full participation in the call
- If the patient has a new concern or something else causing a mental distraction, offer to listen to the patient discuss the situation
- If the patient does not want to discuss the situation, offer to reschedule the call for later in the week

CASE STUDY FOR COMMUNICATION

Doreen is a nurse working for New Age Health Care, a health insurance company. In this capacity, Doreen is responsible for calling a panel of enrollees to discuss their health promotion/disease prevention activities. Doreen has a list of all approved benefits per enrollee and needs to contact 20 enrollees per day.

Doreen works in a call center with 125 other nurses. Each nurse has a cubicle measuring 4 feet by 2 feet. The cubicle walls extend 2 feet up from the desktop. The nurse sitting opposite from Doreen is tall and her head can be seen above the top of the cubicle wall.

On Monday, Doreen comes to work and opens up her assigned enrollees list for the day. She notices that of the 20 enrollees 15 are new to the program. This means Doreen will have to introduce the program to the enrollee, answer any questions, and end the call with the enrollee agreeing to participate in the program.

The first enrollee that Doreen contacted did not answer the telephone so she left a message asking for the enrollee to return the call as soon as possible.

Reflect and answer the following questions:

- Was it appropriate for Doreen to leave a message asking the enrollee to return the call as soon as possible?
- Did Doreen effectively communicate the purpose of making the call?

Later in the morning, Doreen asks to speak to an enrollee; however, the person who answered the call will not give the telephone to the enrollee but rather repeats everything Doreen says to the enrollee. Doreen can hear the enrollee talking and asking questions that are repeated by the person taking the call.

- Is this an effective method to communicate with the enrollee?
- What challenges or hazards exist when using this communication method?

It's the end of the day, and Doreen is placing her last call. This enrollee is very concerned about a health problem and asks Doreen many questions about it. Doreen suggests that the enrollee make an appointment to see the primary health care provider, but the enrollee hesitates because of the cost of co-pays. The enrollee says that the health problem has been going on for months and if it were serious, she would have died by now.

- What statements should Doreen use to respond to this enrollee's health concern?
- What responsibility do you think Doreen has to report the health concern to the health plan?

CASE STUDY FOR ACTIVE LISTENING

Anita works in a call center located in an urban office building. The organization provides disease management and health promotion care to patients with a variety of chronic illnesses. Anita has a case load of patients to contact every day and notices that only two new names are on the list.

After placing the first call, the person who answered the telephone asks Anita to wait and places the phone down. Anita hears a dog barking in the background. Several other voices can be heard discussing plans for after-school activities and requesting money for lunch. Anita hears all of this conversation and gently begins to say "hello, hello" into the telephone. There is no response, but the activities occurring in the patient's home continue. After a few minutes, someone picks up the phone and says "hello?" Anita introduces herself, the program, and begins the call to have the patient become engaged in the process. As the patient is responding, a loud bang is heard.

- What should Anita do?
- Was it appropriate for Anita to stay on the line and listen to the activities and conversation occurring in the patient's home?

The patient is stunned by the noise and asks Anita to hold on and the phone is again placed down. Anita hears someone shouting and now a scream and cries can be heard. In a few seconds, Anita hears someone say "you are alright; the noise is what scared you" and then the patient returns to the telephone. Anita resumes the conversation and asks the patient to validate personal identity. The patient says "wait a minute" and is heard shouting to someone to close the front door and don't forget to "pick up your little sister after school." The patient returns and says "it's just so hectic here in the mornings."

- If you were Anita, would you continue the call?
- What could be done to minimize the patient's distractions during future calls?

KEY POINTS

- A myriad of situations can occur when providing telephonic patient/client care.
- Traditional techniques used to assess a patient/client need to be altered when applying them to telenursing.
- The major tools used in telenursing are communication and active listening.
- These skills need to be sharpened and finely tuned when providing telenursing care.

CHAPTER 3

Professional Preparation for Telehealth Nursing

LEARNING OUTCOMES

Upon completion of this chapter, the nurse will:

1. Summarize suggested experience to perform telephonic patient/ client care
2. Discuss licensure considerations
3. Examine the changes that have occurred in the credentialing examination

RECOMMENDED EXPERIENCE

Most organizations that advertise for telenursing positions ask for a minimum of 1 year of direct hands-on clinical experience. Some organizations ask for 3 to 5 years, depending on the health problems of the patients/clients to be contacted. The type of experience, though, is important to note. The vast majority of patients who will be receiving telenursing care are middle-aged to older adults. Because of this, the nurse should have experience caring for adults with some type or form of chronic illness.

Experience should be in medical–surgical or geriatric nursing. Nurses who have worked in intensive care areas or surgical suites and postanesthesia care areas might be interested in the telenursing role; however, their experience communicating and teaching patients about long-term health promotion and preventive actions may be limited.

The experience that most closely relates to telephonic nursing is community or public health services provided through home care. Nurses who have worked extensively with patients or clients who are not hospitalized have had opportunities to master communication skills and provide wellness/disease management teaching.

At times, an employer or health insurance agency contracts or hires nurses to provide telephonic care to employees or enrollees. In these situations, the age of the patient may be less than middle age, and there is a chance that the patient may be a child. Because of this, many telenursing providers will have on staff a few nurses with pediatric experience. Keep in mind, though, when providing telenursing care to a minor, communication will most likely occur through the parent or legal guardian. The ability to effectively communicate with an adult is essential.

The nurse desiring a telenursing role should have expert or outstanding verbal and written communication skills. This includes the ability to problem-solve and troubleshoot health care questions, issues, and patient concerns. During the course of a routine care call, the patient may ask a question about another health issue that is not documented or has just manifested. The nurse must have the flexibility to change the course of the call in order to meet the patient's needs.

When initially contacting a patient for telenursing care, most of the first encounter will be invested in data collection. Depending on the sponsoring organization, the nurse may need to follow a specific set of questions or criteria to determine the patient's eligibility to participate. For example, a patient may have had a routine serum glucose level drawn as part of an electrolyte panel during a recent health care provider office visit. The health insurance plan receives a notice of billing to pay for the laboratory services, and health plan software tagged the serum glucose as a test that was performed. According to the health plan's algorithm for patient selection, a serum glucose level is used when caring for patients with diabetes. The patient is then identified as being a member of the diabetes disease management program. When the nurse places the first call to the patient, one of the eligibility questions might be "how long have you been diagnosed with diabetes?" At this point, the patient may respond with a certain number of years or adamantly deny having the diagnosis. If the patient has not been diagnosed with diabetes, they are deemed ineligible for the program and would be deleted from the nurse's future care call panel.

It is important for the nurse to recognize "teachable moments" throughout the assessment process. For example, the nurse learns that a patient with diabetes works in a home garden as a primary leisure activity. The nurse should deviate from the assessment or criteria and ask the patient what type of footwear and gloves are worn while gardening because it is important for the patient to avoid cuts and scrapes to either the hands or feet. From here, the nurse can then redirect the call back to the original assessment/criteria process.

One of the major issues identified by patients who receive telenursing care is the amount of time spent assessing is far greater than receiving any valuable teaching. In other words, the nurse is to do more than collect data. The data are to be used to provide care to address the patient's needs or support health promotion activities. Nurses might be overheard going through a list of assessment questions, sounding like they are reading from a script. This approach is not welcoming or inviting, and the patient may choose to not participate in the future.

TELENURSING SCOPE OF PRACTICE

In 1995, the American Academy of Ambulatory Care Nursing (AAACN) decided that telephonic patient/client care was a subspecialty of ambulatory care. After careful study, this organization published the first set of telenursing standards in 2001. Subsequently, these standards were reviewed and updated with the most recent revision published in 2011.

The standards of practice for professional telehealth nursing are divided into two domains: standards of clinical practice and standards of professional performance.

Standards of Clinical Practice

The standards of clinical practice are aligned with the nursing process and include:

- *Assessment:* Systematically collect data related to health needs/concerns of a patient, group, or population
- *Nursing diagnosis:* Analyze assessed data to identify diagnoses applicable for health promotion, health maintenance, or to address health-related concerns
- *Identification of expected outcomes/goals:* Identify outcomes for an individualized plan of care for a patient, group, or population
- *Planning:* Identify strategies or approaches to achieve expected outcomes or goals
- *Implementation:* Perform actions to achieve expected outcomes/goals
- *Evaluation:* Determine amount of progress toward the achievement of outcomes

Implementation is further subdivided into the following substandards:

- *Coordination of care:* Serve as the point of contact within and among practice settings
- *Health teaching and health promotion:* Implement strategies to promote wellness
- *Consultation:* Facilitate actions with other health care providers to effectively change the patient, group, or population's health

Standards of Professional Performance

The standards of professional performance identify professional and organizational behaviors and include:

- *Ethics:* Ensure patient/client, group, population rights in all areas of practice
- *Education:* Actively maintain knowledge and competency to reflect current nursing practice
- *Research and evidence-based practice:* Incorporate best practices to promote continuous quality improvement and advance the practice of telenursing
- *Performance improvement:* Enhance telecommunication practices
- *Communication:* Implement a variety of approaches to support the nurse–patient/client relationship and build professional relationships across the health care continuum
- *Leadership:* Attain and implement leadership skills to enhance health care of patients, groups, and the population
- *Collaboration:* Interact with patients, families, groups, populations, caregivers, and other health care professionals when delivering telenursing care
- *Professional practice evaluation:* Ongoing review of professional practice as it relates to organizational expectations, position expectations, professional standards, and regulatory bodies
- *Resource utilization:* Implement fiscally responsible strategies when providing telenursing
- *Environment:* Perform work in a safe, efficient, hazard-free, and ergonomically correct setting

LICENSURE AND CREDENTIALING

Licensure

Licensure beyond an RN is not required to practice telephonic patient/client care. One issue with licensure, however, has to do with the state of the nurse's license and the location of the patient.

If a telephonic nurse is contacting a patient/client in a state in which the nurse currently has a license to practice, there is no issue. But, if the patient lives in a state that is different from the nurse's licensed state, the nurse will need to obtain a license to practice nursing in that state.

Licensure becomes complicated if the nurse's state of residence is a member of the Nurse Licensure Compact. The Nurse Licensure Compact is legislation that acknowledges nursing state license reciprocity. If the nurse resides in a state that is a member of the Nurse Licensure Compact, that nurse can relocate to another state with the compact and not need to obtain another state license to practice.

For the telephonic nurse:

- If the nurse and patient/client both reside in states that are members of the Nurse Licensure Compact, an additional state license is not required.
- If the nurse resides in a state within the Nurse Licensure Compact and the patient does not, the nurse needs to obtain a license to practice in the patient's state.
- If the patient resides in a state that is within the Nurse Licensure Compact but the nurse does not, the nurse needs to obtain a license to contact the patient.

States that are current members of the Nurse Licensure Compact are:

- Arizona
- Arkansas
- Colorado
- Delaware
- Idaho
- Iowa
- Kentucky

- Maine
- Maryland
- Mississippi
- Missouri
- Montana
- Nebraska
- New Hampshire

- New Mexico
- North Carolina
- North Dakota
- Rhode Island
- South Carolina
- South Dakota

- Tennessee
- Texas
- Utah
- Virginia
- Wisconsin

It is best to find out from your hiring organization if an additional state license is required before placing any patient calls.

Credentialing

For many years, nurses could become certified in telenursing through the National Certification Corporate (NCC). However, this certification examination was discontinued December 31, 2007. Any nurse who is currently certified through the NCC would need to continue to meet NCC's recertification requirements.

Because the NCC recognized the AAACN as being the leader for telenursing, content on telenursing became a part of the AAACN ambulatory care certification examination in 2009. The primary reason for this certification change was because the telephonic nurse provides care to the patient or client in the "ambulatory" setting—the home. This certification examination is offered by the American Nursing Credentialing Center (ANCC). Please note that certification as an ambulatory care nurse has not been made a mandatory requirement by hiring organizations.

KEY POINTS

- There is not one set of criteria to practice as a telephonic nurse.
- Nurses with experience in home care and providing care to adults or geriatric patients/clients would have the best previous experience for the role.
- Be aware of state licensure issues that affect the nurse's state of residence and potential patients'/clients' states of residence.
- Certification as a telephonic nurse is available through the ANCC. Most organizations do not require certification for employment.

BIBLIOGRAPHY

American Academy of Ambulatory Care Nursing. (2011). *Scope and standards of practice for professional telehealth nursing* (5th ed.). Pitman, NJ: Author.

Hughes, R. G. (2008). Patient safety, telenursing, and telehealth. In *Patient safety and quality: An evidence-based handbook for nurses* (chap. 48). Rockville, MD: Agency for Healthcare Research and Quality.

National Council of State Boards of Nursing. (2015). Nurse licensure compact. Retrieved from https://www.ncsbn.org/nurse-licensure-compact .htm

CHAPTER 4

Patient/Client Perspective on Telehealth Nursing

LEARNING OUTCOMES

Upon completion of this chapter, the nurse will:

1. Summarize the methods in which patients/clients are identified to participate in telenursing care
2. Recognize barriers for patient/client participation in a telephonic nursing care program
3. Strategize approaches to overcome patient/client barriers to participation in a telephonic nursing care program
4. Examine the importance of confidentiality and adherence to Health Insurance Portability and Accountability Act (HIPAA) legislation when providing telephonic patient/client care

PATIENT/CLIENT IDENTIFICATION

Nurses who work in telenursing will not be "looking for" or "finding" clients. Patients (or in some situations, clients or enrollees) will be provided from contracts with health care providers or employers. The contracting organization will most likely provide the individual's:

- Name
- Address
- Telephone number
- Health issue/concern

It is on the health issue or concern that the nurse will focus when contacting the client. Before making the first contact, the nurse needs to become familiar with the information provided. For example, if a client has been repeatedly hospitalized for infections, the nurse may have access to information from his or her:

- Hospitalization
- Laboratory results
- Diagnostic test results
- Prescribed medications
- Activity status
- Diet
- Prescribed treatment

The purpose for being enrolled in the telenursing program must be identified. If the intention is to prevent hospitalization or rehospitalization, documentation should be provided about the health concern. The nurse needs as much information as possible about the health problem before making the first telephone call.

Another scenario would be clients who have a chronic health problem. The health plan likely identified the individual as someone who would benefit from counseling or teaching telephone calls. The intention here would be to discuss:

- The chronic health problem
- Adherence with prescribed medications and treatments
- Frequency of follow-up examinations with the health care provider
- Actions to reduce exacerbations of the chronic health issue
- Additional ways to manage the chronic health issue

The last possible scenario for patient participation would be an employer-sponsored wellness program. In this situation, the individual would not be referred to as "patient" but rather as an "enrollee" or "participant."

Individuals enrolled through an employee-sponsored program may be offered a list of services all designed to improve the employee's health. Examples of services offered include:

- Smoking cessation
- Weight management
- Stress management
- Participation in physical activity

The employer may decide which teaching materials, websites, or agencies to use for the services. If this is the case, the nurse will need access to these items in order to conduct an effective telenursing call.

IDENTIFYING BARRIERS

In an ideal world, every client who is contacted telephonically by a nurse will be eager to talk and find value in the conversation. Unfortunately, this is not always the case. The bad news is the patient may immediately hang up. The good news is the first call is often the most difficult to complete.

Oftentimes, the first questions that a potential patient or participant will ask are:

● How did you get my phone number?
● Why are you calling me?

People are naturally skeptical of receiving any telephone communication if it is concerning personal health information. Consider yourself fortunate if the person does not immediately hang up. There is a window of opportunity here where the nurse can engage the person and gain support and cooperation.

Another issue that potential patients will have is the cost. Patients will immediately think that you are "trying to sell" them something. It is essential to know how the patients are identified for the organization in which you are providing telenursing care and how the care is being paid for.

Patients will also be concerned about the amount of time each of the telephone calls is going to take. Today people are very busy. Depending on the age and health problem, a patient may be working, caring for children, or supporting aging family members. Time can be as important to someone as cost.

OVERCOMING BARRIERS

A variety of strategies can be used when faced with patient/client engagement challenges. These strategies may be interchangeable but have been divided according to patient situation.

Patient/Client Who Was Previously Hospitalized

A cold call to a recently discharged patient is probably the least difficult one to make. The patient may have been informed that follow-up phone calls can occur and be provided by the hospital or health care provider. However, the patient might not expect a telephone call from the health insurance plan. Explaining how the health insurance plan has gotten involved might be the greatest challenge.

When placing a call to a recently hospitalized patient, keep the following in mind:

- The patient is recovering from an illness or exacerbation. They might be easily fatigued with talking on the telephone.
- The patient may be starting new medication and not totally aware of the actions, purpose, and expected effects. You might be doing quite a bit of medication teaching.
- The patient might be expecting or receiving home care. A challenge might be explaining the different roles and the importance of the patient's participation in both.
- The patient might be "turned off" from so much talk about illnesses that they just do not want to be bothered. You might be challenged with persuading them that the calls will help prevent hospitalizations for the same or similar problem in the future.

For the recently hospitalized patient, the first telephone call might be referred to as a posthospitalization call. Besides validating the patient's demographic information, telephone number, and best time to call, the actual work of the call focuses on the reason for the hospitalization and the plans for care and recovery at home. Things to keep in mind when engaging with a patient recently hospitalized include:

- The length of this telephone call might be 20 to 30 minutes.
- Do not rush the patient.
- Follow the patient's lead. If the patient wants to talk about the illness for a short while encourage them to do so. Gently guide the patient away from the hospitalization and refocus on actions that can be taken to prevent additional hospital care in the future.
- Ask about support in the home environment.

- Be sure that the patient has had all posthospitalization medication prescriptions filled.
- Find out if follow-up care needs have been met or obtained such as home oxygen, sleep apnea devices, hospital bed, and assistive devices.
- Conduct a home safety assessment to include safety in the kitchen and bathroom and if all smoke detectors have been checked with fully charged batteries.

Patient/Client With a Chronic Illness

Health plans follow or track expenses by enrollees for specific health issues. Individuals who repeatedly use health plan benefits may be "red flagged" for a disease management program. A disease management program is one in which specific actions or interventions are used to ensure that the particular "disease" is managed appropriately. Some of the most frequently created disease management programs include:

- Diabetes
- Chronic obstructive lung/pulmonary disease (COLD/COPD)
- Asthma
- Back pain
- Heart failure
- Coronary artery disease
- Stroke
- Arthritis
- Cancer
- HIV/AIDS
- Gastroesophageal reflux disease (GERD)
- Hypertension
- Irritable bowel syndrome (IBS)

When contacting a patient to participate in a disease management program, the contracting organization will most likely ask for specific information to collect during the first call. This is oftentimes done to ensure that the enrollee truly belongs in the program. For example:

- The health plan flags that a patient has had repeated blood glucose testing completed and immediately places the patient into the diabetes management program. When asking how many years the patient has been treated for diabetes, the patient may respond with the number of years or argue that diabetes has never been diagnosed.

● The health plan flags a patient after having a breast biopsy to be placed in the cancer disease management program. The nurse may learn from the patient that the biopsy was negative and the patient does not belong in the program or the patient is scheduled for surgery and further treatment in which case the patient referral to the program is legitimate.

Providing telephone care to a patient with a chronic health problem can be challenging. The patient may not want to talk about the health problem or feel that the care currently receiving from health care providers is sufficient. The nurse may need to spend additional time convincing the patient about the value of participating in the program and urge them to continue for at least a short while before making a decision to opt out.

Patient/Client Enrolled in a Wellness Program

Wellness programs were once all the rage in the early 2000s. Many employers viewed these programs as a way to keep the workforce healthy and reduce the risk of chronic disease development. Many of these programs were linked to employees' health insurance coverage and helped to determine the amount of payment that the employee had to contribute for coverage. Actions that linked participation in the wellness program with health insurance coverage contribution included:

● Blood glucose levels
● Lipid panel
● Current weight
● Participation in a weight reduction/management program (if applicable)
● Proof of smoking cessation
● Documentation of attending sessions at a local gym

Although employer-based programs still exist, many health plans have changed the approach. With the signing of the Affordable Care Act (ACE) in 2009, employers may choose to use web-based wellness applications instead of live nursing calls. In some situations, the first preliminary steps are completed by the employee online. Depending upon the information provided, the employee may not need telephonic nursing care. In other situations, the employee may qualify for a telephonic nursing call once a month or a few times a year.

The goal for employee-based programs is to ensure a healthy workforce and reduce the amount and cost for health care in efforts to keep the employer's contribution for health care premiums at the lowest possible level. These types of programs have had different degrees of acceptance:

- Employees feel this is a violation of personal health information and resent having an employer dictate actions and behaviors when not at work
- Employees feel that is an added benefit provided by the employing organization and fully participate in order to save money

The first telephone call to participate in a wellness program is probably the most challenging for the telephonic nurse. Beyond the expected level of skepticism, the participant may want to know:

- How much information does the employer have about the employee's health?
- Who gave the employer permission to have information about the employee's health?
- Will issues with health cause the employer to terminate the employee?
- How can the employer be trusted not to terminate the employee in the future?
- Who does the telephonic nurse work for? The employer or the health plan?
- What will happen if the employee refuses to participate?
- What happens to this information if the employee chooses to quit the current position?
- How will this information affect the cost of health care premiums in the future?

Wellness activities are not always in the forefront of people's minds. Most people understand that eating a healthy diet, participating in activity, and not smoking are important for long-term health; however, not all people realize that actions can be taken nearly every day to help ensure health. Responses by individuals targeted for participation in an employee wellness program may include:

- I have never been hospitalized so why do I need this?
- I am not overweight and I don't smoke so this isn't for me.
- I'm too busy to spend time talking to someone about something that I already know.
- This is just another way for my employer to control me and I don't want to have anything to do with it.
- I get a flu shot and see my doctor once a year. What can you possibly tell me that my own doctor hasn't already?

It is easy to become frustrated with the participant's questions and lack of interest. The goal here is to at least have the employee "think about" participating and then follow up again in a few weeks. Preventing the participant from opting out may be as important as fully engaging them in the program.

CONFIDENTIALITY

Confidentiality is a big news topic. People hear on the television almost daily how health plan enrollee data have been hacked or private information about health status has been breached. Federal investigations are ongoing and people become very scared—and rightly so. In other situations, entire identities have been stolen. Recovering from having a stolen identity can take months or even years. It is easy to understand why someone would hesitate to talk to someone if they don't know about the person's health or personal care needs.

The contracting organization must have plans and processes in place to ensure that the personal information about the enrollees is secure. Any third-party organization hired to provide telenursing care must comply with the contracting organization's expectations for confidentiality. Nurses hired for telenursing positions have to complete a rigorous interview process and have documentation of ethical behavior. But this may mean nothing to the patient on the other end of the telephone line.

Nurses providing telephonic care are challenged with having to verbally prove that each conversation and contents of the telephone calls will be held in the strictest confidence. Actions to help allay any patient's anxieties about confidentiality include:

- Providing the patient with your full name
- Providing the patient with the location of the business
- Providing the patient with the telephone number of the employing agency
- Encouraging the patient to call into the employing agency at any time
- Not asking for the patient's social security number or credit card information because this information is not used or required

Some telephonic nursing companies have telephone systems that automatically "record calls for quality purposes." It is essential that this information be shared with every patient before getting into the specifics about the call. The patient must understand that although the call is recorded, the purpose is to measure and evaluate the nurse's performance and not judge the patient's responses, health issues, or care concerns.

Patients may also worry about the information getting into "the wrong hands." You may find yourself explaining about the employing agency's computer system, log-ins, backups, and encryption software. Although this type of information may be well beyond the average nurse's comprehension and practice, taking a few extra minutes to calm a patient's anxieties will help in the development of the therapeutic relationship and aid in the achievement of the purpose of the current and future calls.

HIPAA REGULATIONS

The HIPAA was passed in 1996 and continues to be reviewed and revised today. The original act had three areas:

- Privacy rules
- Security rules
- Administrative controls/enforcement rules

Privacy Rules

Privacy focuses on the use and disclosure of personal/protected health information (PHI). According to this rule, PHI is to be protected and shared only to provide or promote high-quality care. In telenursing, the sharing of PHI occurs from the health plan, to the nurse's employing organization, and back to the health plan. Information is not shared with other third-party vendors, hospitals, or employers.

Hard copy personal health information is not a practice in telenursing. Communication occurs via the telephone and documentation is placed directly into a software application. There is no reason to have a "medical record" or "file" for any patient enrolled in a telephonic nursing program.

Some telephonic nursing agencies might generate "calling lists" for special telephone campaigns. Examples of special campaigns include reminding patients in September or October to get an annual flu inoculation or telephoning patients with diabetes to obtain a hemoglobin A1c level every 3 months. These lists rarely provide information beyond the patient's name and telephone number. Nursing staff still access the patient's information in the computer software and document information about the call there.

At the conclusion of special "campaigns," any hard copy information with patient identification (name, telephone number) is destroyed through the use of paper shredders or via contract with an agency that specifically destroys personal health information.

Security Rules

The security rules are those written to ensure that PHI electronically collected and documented is secure. This means that anyone who is entering or viewing PHI has the right credentials to do so. Additional characteristics of the security rules include:

- Each nurse has an individual log-in
- Each log-in is password protected
- Nurses sign forms stating that log-ins and passwords are not shared
- Software used for PHI is encrypted (cannot be breached or hacked)

Business associate agreements exist between the telenursing organization and other organizations that may be involved with the backup and storage of PHI. The purpose of these agreements is to expect the third-party agency to protect the PHI and ensure for its security. As of this writing there have been no data or breaches of PHI from any telenursing organization.

Administrative Controls/Enforcement Rules

The administrative controls/enforcement rules focus on actions to take if a breach of PHI occurs. Breaches can be costly to both the individual who caused the breach and the employing organization.

HITECH ACT

Just when many health care organizations mastered the expectations of HIPAA, another major piece of legislation was passed. The Health Information Technology for Economic and Clinical Health Act (HITECH Act) was created in 2009 as an incentive for health care providers to adopt the use of electronic health records (EHRs). Through this act, health care providers were provided with incentives to demonstrate meaningful use of the EHR. This act does not impact telenursing practice.

EXERCISES TO IMPROVE PATIENT/CLIENT ENGAGEMENT

Because for many nurses this is a new way of providing patient care, an opportunity to practice without having a "live" patient on the telephone might be beneficial. It is always best to perform these exercises with two people participating.

EXERCISE 1: POSTHOSPITALIZATION PATIENT/CLIENT

Arrange two chairs back to back so that it is not possible for one person to see the other. One person will play the role of the nurse and the other, the patient. Use the following script for this exercise:

Nurse	Patient/Client
(The telephone is ringing and picked up.)	
	Hello?
Hello. My name is John Williams and I am a nurse with Blue Spruce Health Plan. Is Mr. Wainwright available?	
	That's me. What do you want?
Well, Mr. Wainwright, your health plan, Blue Spruce, has contracted with us to give you a call since you just got out of the hospital.	
	How do you know I was in the hospital? Who told you that?
Well, your health plan, Blue Spruce, asked for a nurse to give you call since you've been discharged. Are you saying that you weren't in the hospital?	
	Oh, I was but I just wanted to know how you knew I was since I have no idea who you are or why you are calling me.
As a part of your health plan benefits, calls are made to all patients once they are discharged from the hospital. The purpose of the calls is to follow up with you to make sure that you are recovering and have everything that you need so you don't end up in the hospital again.	
	Well there's no guarantee I won't need to go back in the hospital but it won't be for this problem.
Before we go any further Mr. Wainwright, can I ask if you would verify your home address?	

(continued)

(*continued*)

Nurse	Patient/Client
	No, you tell me what my address is and I'll tell you if it's right or not.
Okay. I have you residing at 922 Greenbush Drive in Bend, Oregon.	
	That's right.
And is this the best telephone number to reach you?	
	Yes. I don't have one of those cell phone things. I'm too old to try to learn how to use one of them.
One more question, Mr. Wainwright. Can you verify your birthday, month and year only.	
	You tell me …
January 1931	
	That's right.
Thank you. As a level of security I need to tell you that this call may be recorded for quality purposes only.	
	What are they going to be listening for?
It's to make sure that I'm providing the right care to you.	
	That's okay.
Okay, great. Mr. Wainwright, can you tell me why you were hospitalized?	
	I thought you knew that already.
I have some information but it's always helpful to hear the patient say it in his own words.	
	I had some pretty bad stomach pain and needed surgery to fix something with my bowels.

(*continued*)

(*continued*)

Nurse	Patient/Client
How are you feeling now?	
	Well, I'm pretty sore and I can't do a lot, like lift things that weigh more than 5 pounds, but I'm doing a whole lot better than I was a few days ago.
That's good to hear. Mr. Wainwright, do you have the time now to go over your medicines and other care your surgeon has prescribed for you?	
	Sure.
(The call continues with the nurse fully engaging the posthospitalization patient.)	

This exercise had a positive outcome. What strategies could the nurse have used if the patient wasn't willing to participate?

EXERCISE 2: DISEASE MANAGEMENT PATIENT

Using the same chair arrangement, identify one person to play the nurse and the other to play the patient. The script for this exercise is as follows:

Nurse	Patient/Client
(Telephone ringing ...)	
	Hello?
Hello! I'm James with AmeriHealth. Is Linda Williams available?	

(*continued*)

(*continued*)

Nurse	Patient/Client
	This is Linda. Why are you calling?
Ms. Williams, as I mentioned, I'm a nurse with AmeriHealth. Your health plan has identified you as someone who would benefit from receiving telephone calls for your chronic health problem.	
	What chronic health problem?
Are you saying that you haven't been diagnosed with a chronic health problem?	
	What's that? I mean I have arthritis but it's something I live with every day. I don't consider that chronic. I'm not sick.
Have you been to see your doctor recently or any other health care provider?	
	Last week I had a doctor's appointment and he sent me for x-rays and blood tests before he would call a prescription in to the drugstore. But I'm not sick. I still work and everything.
This program is designed to help keep you as healthy as possible with your arthritis.	
	You mean you're going to help me stay healthy and work even though I've got pain in both my hips and knees? I don't think so.
Have you been seeing your doctor for this health problem for very long?	
	A few years. I just don't see how you are going to help me.

(*continued*)

(*continued*)

Nurse	Patient/Client
Besides the medication have you made any other changes in your life because of the arthritis pain?	
	You mean cutting down on the number of times I go up and down the steps and not being able to go for walks anymore so that I've gained 10 pounds over the last 3 months? Yeah, who needs those kinds of changes?
It sounds like the arthritis is getting in the way of your regular activity.	
	To say the least.
Well with my phone calls I might be able to help you manage your weight a little better and help you increase your activity so that the pain won't get in the way so much.	
	If you could do that then it would be worth it.
Okay then. But before we go any further there are a few housekeeping things that need to be done.	
	Okay.
(The call continues with the nurse validating the patient's identity and explaining that the call could be recorded for monitoring purposes.)	

In this situation, the nurse immediately engaged the patient to discuss the impact of the chronic illness on the patient's life. This was done before validating the patient's identity and best time to call. Although not ideal it is an approach to help engage the patient to participate in the program.

EXERCISE 3: WELLNESS PROGRAM PARTICIPANT

This final exercise provides an example of a conversation to engage a participant in a wellness program. The same chair arrangement should be used with other people playing the role of the nurse and participant.

Nurse	Patient/Client
(The phone is ringing.)	
	Yeah, hello.
Hello. This is Bob calling from Sun Valley Health. Is Jeff available?	
	I'm Jeff. Who are you with?
Sun Valley Health.	
	Never heard of them. You have the right person?
Sun Valley Health is a wellness agency. We provide wellness programs to employees of organizations who have purchased the benefit for their employees.	
	So you're telling me my employer told you to call me? What's this about?
Your employer has purchased a wellness benefit for all employees. What we do is call the employee and talk with them about different ways to stay healthy.	
	Funny. I can't get a raise but my employer has money for this.

(continued)

(*continued*)

Nurse	Patient/Client
I can't address the cost or reasons why your employer purchased this benefit. What I can do is talk with you about the different approaches available to keep you healthy.	
	I haven't taken a sick day for years. Why all of a sudden I'm getting calls about my health?
Have you not received any information from your employer about this benefit?	
	There was some meeting about benefits a month or so ago but I had to work on an emergency report and I missed it. So what do I need to do?
Well, I need to tell you more about the program and the different approaches. But first I have to make sure I'm talking to the right person.	
	You already know my name what else do you have to do?
(The nurse continues with validating the participant's identity and potential recording of the call for quality purposes before discussing the program elements.)	

Individuals enrolled in wellness programs through an employer may have negative comments about the cost and the hidden "agenda" for enrollment. Stay neutral when negative comments are made about an employer. Your role is to introduce the program and provide approaches to maintain health and wellness and not engage or encourage any employer bashing.

KEY POINTS

- Individuals are referred for telenursing care through a health plan or employer.
- Patients discharged from the hospital and those who are frequent users of health benefits most likely will be referred to a telenursing organization by the health plan.
- Participants in wellness programs most likely will be listed or included for contact through an employer.
- All people will not want to participate in the program. There will be excuses and barriers.
- There are many approaches to overcome the barriers to participation.
- At all times be aware of potential issues with confidentiality.
- Adhere to your organization's HIPAA policies and procedures.

BIBLIOGRAPHY

U.S. Department of Health and Human Services. (2016). Health information privacy. Retrieved from http://www.hhs.gov/hipaa

Introduction to Body Systems

The assessment of a patient or client through the use of a telephone is a new experience for many nurses. As earlier chapters have emphasized, you will not be able to observe or touch the patient/client to determine firsthand what might be occurring. Careful and thoughtful questioning will be used to collect as much data as possible.

This section focuses on the major body systems, outlining approaches telehealth nurses use in conducting an assessment. Each chapter begins with a brief review of anatomy and then provides questions for use in assessing the body system. Tips and techniques are provided where appropriate, along with practice scenarios that you can use to work through potential client interactions.

CHAPTER 5

Integumentary System

Upon completion of this chapter, the nurse will:

1. Outline the areas to include when assessing the integumentary system
2. Identify appropriate questions to assess the integumentary system
3. Analyze care to address health problems of the integumentary system

THE INTEGUMENTARY SYSTEM

The Skin

During our education, nurses learn that the skin is the largest organ of the body and is viewed as the first line of defense against illness or diseases. Although this is not an anatomy text, it might be helpful to review a few essential areas about the skin before diving into the assessment.

The skin has two layers: the epidermis and the dermis. The epidermis is the outermost layer and is made up of both dead and living cells. Dead cells are sloughed off and replaced by new cells formed within the innermost layer of the epidermis that contain keratin and melanin. The dermis is the layer that contains the blood vessels, connective tissue, and sebaceous glands. Some of the hair follicles are in this layer. Under the dermis is a layer of subcutaneous tissue. Here the rest of the hair follicles, sweat glands, and fat are stored.

The skin serves several functions:

- Controls temperature (or thermoregulation)
- Serves as a barrier to contain all body fluids

- Prevents harmful microorganisms from entering body tissues
- Serves as a sensory organ for touch and temperature
- Excretes harmful substances through sweat glands
- Synthesizes vitamin D from ultraviolet light

Hair and Nails

The hair and nails are considered appendage structures of the skin. Hair follicles are over most of the total body surface except for the soles of the feet and palms of the hands. The nails are at the end of the fingers and toes.

ASSESSMENT OVERVIEW

The skin assessment is one of the most challenging to assess when providing telenursing care.

- You will not be able to see or touch the client's skin
- Rashes and skin temperature will need to be described
- Skin turgor cannot be directly assessed
- Wound size will not be directly measured
- Drainage cannot be assessed for characteristics and odor

The assessment of this major body system will be very creative, and it can be quite lengthy. When discussing the integumentary system with your patient over the telephone, determine first if the patient is experiencing any particular skin problem. If so, focus on that area first. If not, complete a general assessment of the skin, hair, and nails.

QUESTIONS TO ASSESS THE INTEGUMENTARY SYSTEM

Skin	
Component	**Question**
General	Describe your skin.
Texture	How does it feel? Dry or moist?

(continued)

(continued)

Skin	
Component	**Question**
	Are there any areas where the texture of your skin is different? For example: at the elbows, the knees, the nape of the neck, upper back, and over the buttocks
	How does the skin feel over these areas? Drier? Scaling? Itchy?
	How long have these changes been occurring over the different skin areas?
	Describe the color of your skin.
	Has the color of your skin changed at all over the last few months?
	If the color has changed, what is the change?
	Name the areas where the change in skin color has occurred.
Rashes	Do you have any rashes on your skin?
	Where are they located?
	How long have you had the rash?
	Explain how the rash appears.
	Does the rash have a pattern?
	Are the areas round?
	Do the areas "run together" as one large patch?
	Are the areas small and separated by large patches of skin?
	Are the areas grouped together, for example, on the front of the lower leg or the outer area of the upper thigh?
	Does the rash form a straight line?
	Does the rash include blisters?
	Is there any fluid coming out of the rash areas?
	Does the rash itch?

(continued)

(continued)

Skin	
Component	**Question**
	What have you been using to help with the rash? Does it help?
	Have you talked with your doctor or health care provider about the rash?
Moisture	In your own words, describe how much you sweat.
	In what areas does this sweating occur the most? For example, under the armpits, the neck, around the face, the groin, behind the knees.
	Has the amount that you sweat changed over the last weeks or months?
	Is there an odor associated with the sweat?
	Have you noticed if the sweating is more or less during a particular time of the day or night?
	Do you have a history of skin rashes or allergies?
Integrity	Do you have any areas where the skin is eroded, scaled, peeling, or blistered?
	Are you experiencing any drainage from skin areas?
	Do you have any sores, ulcers, or wounds on your skin? Where are these areas located?
	Describe what the sore/ulcer/wound looks like.
	Describe what the skin around the sore/ulcer/wound looks like.
	Is the skin around the sore/ulcer/wound warm/hot to the touch? Red or pale in color?
	What have you been doing to treat the sore/ulcer/ wound?
	Have you talked with your doctor or health care provider about the sore/ulcer/wound?
	Is the treatment improving the sore/ulcer/wound?
	Do you have any skin tags or moles?

(continued)

(continued)

Skin	
Component	**Question**
	Where are these located?
	Are there any body areas that have more skin tags or moles?
	Have you noticed any changes to these areas?
	Have you had these areas examined by a doctor, health care provider, or dermatologist?
	Have you had any skin tags/moles treated?
	Have you ever been diagnosed or treated for skin cancer?
	If so, what was the location on your body that the skin tags/moles were treated?
	Are you taking or prescribed any medication to treat a particular skin problem? • If so, what is the skin problem? • What is the name of the medication? • How often do you apply it? • How long are you supposed to use it? • What follow-up has your doctor or health care provider prescribed for the skin problem?
	Do you have any lumps?
	Where are these located?
	If lumps are present, how do they feel? • Hard? Soft? • Can they be moved under the skin or are they firmly attached? • What is the color of the skin over the lump? • Is the lump itchy? • Red or warm to the touch?
	Have you ever had these before? If so, how were they treated?
	Do you have any bumps or swollen areas on the skin?
	Where are these located?
	Do you know how they developed? For example, did you bump the area against a piece of furniture?

(continued)

(continued)

Skin	
Component	**Question**
	Describe the color of the skin over the bump.
	Does the skin feel hot or cool to the touch?
	Have you ever had these before? If so, how were they treated?
	Do you have any bruises on the skin?
	Where are these located?
	Do they have a pattern? Are they clustered together or scattered?
	Are they tender to the touch?
	Describe the color of the bruises.
	Have you ever had these before? If so, how were they treated?
	Do you have any tender or painful areas on the skin?
	Where are these located?
	How long have these areas been tender or painful?
	Have you seen your doctor or health care professional about the lumps, bumps, bruises, or tender/painful areas? • If so, what treatment was prescribed? • Has the treatment improved the area? • Made the area worse? • No noticeable change in the area?
Past history	Have you ever been diagnosed with a problem that specifically affects your skin?
	If so, how was the skin problem treated?
	When was the last time that you experienced the skin problem?
	Does it reoccur at specific times of the year or under specific conditions?
	Have you ever been diagnosed with a skin allergy?
	Have you had any health problems that affected your skin in any way?
	Have you ever taken a medication that caused a skin problem?

(continued)

(*continued*)

Skin	
Component	**Question**
	Do you remember the name of the medication?
	What was the skin problem?
	What was done to treat the skin problem at that time?
	Has that skin problem reoccurred?
	On a scale of 1 to 10 with 1 being worse and 10 being the best, how would you rate your overall skin health at this time?
Bathing, cleansing, basic care	How often do you cleanse the skin? (shower, bathtub, sponge bath)
	What products are used for skin cleansing?
	Do you apply anything on the skin after cleansing it?
	How often do you apply something on the skin through the course of a day? Once, twice, several times?
Sun (UV) exposure	Do you routinely expose your skin to the sun?
	How often do you expose your skin to the sun?
	At what times during the day do you expose your skin to the sun?
	Have you ever used a tanning bed?
	If so, how long was each session?
	How many times did you use the tanning bed?
	Have you ever had a sunburn?
	What did you use to treat the sunburn?
	Do you routinely apply a sunblock when exposing the skin to the sun?
	What sun protection factor (SPF) do you routinely use?
	Have you ever seen a dermatologist for a change in the skin after being exposed to the sun?

(*continued*)

(continued)

Skin	
Component	**Question**
	Have you ever been treated for a sun-related skin change? If so, what was the change and the treatment?
	Have you ever been counseled to avoid exposing your skin to direct sunlight unprotected with a sunblock?
Body Piercings	Do you have any body piercings?
	Where are these piercings located?
	Are you experiencing any swelling, redness, or pain at the areas of the piercings?
Body art	Do you have any tattoos?
	When were the tattoos placed?
	Where are the tattoos located?
	Have you experienced any swelling, redness, or pain at the areas of the tattoos?
	Has the image tattooed changed in any way? Become distorted from swelling?
Hair	
Head	What color is your hair?
	Has your hair changed in color over the last weeks or months?
	How often do you wash your hair?
	How would you describe your hair? Thick, thin, dry, oily, curly, wavy, straight?
	What products do you use on your hair routinely?
	Have you noticed any change in the amount of hair you have on your head?
	When did this change first occur?
	Have you discussed this change in hair on your head with your doctor or health care professional?
	Are you doing anything to address the change in hair on your head?

(continued)

(continued)

Hair	
Component	**Question**
	Are you using any over-the-counter products to increase the amount of hair you have on your head?
	Do you have flakes or dandruff?
	Do you use any products to address the flakes or dandruff?
Body	Have you noticed any changes in the amount of body hair?
	For men: Have you noticed any changes in the amount of facial hair? Do you have any swollen hair follicles on your face that are more noticeable after shaving?
	For women: Have you noticed any changes in the amount of hair under your arms or on your legs? Have you experienced any new facial hair growth?
	For both men and women: Have you discussed this change in body hair with your doctor or health care professional?
Nails	
Fingers	Describe the condition of your fingernails.
	Are your fingernails short or long?
	How do you perform fingernail care? Do you do it yourself or do you go to a nail salon?
	Do you have artificial nails or gels applied to your fingernails?
	Have you had any infections around the nails?
	Have you had any swellings or pain near the cuticle of the nails?
	Describe the shape of your nails.
	Place both of your index fingers together, nail to nail. Can you see a diamond shape of light between the nail surfaces?
	Are your nails straight or curved?
	If they are curved, are the nails growing over the tips of your fingers?
Toes	Describe the condition of your toenails.
	Are your toenails long or short?

(continued)

(*continued*)

Nails	
Component	**Question**
	How do you perform toenail care? Do you go to a podiatrist? Or a salon for routine pedicures?
	What is the color of your toenails?
	Do you routinely have polish or gel applied to your toenails?
	Are any of your toenails crumbling or thickened?
	Do you have any areas of redness/soreness/pain around the toenail or cuticle?

ADDITIONAL QUESTIONS THAT FOCUS ON INTEGUMENTARY HEALTH PROBLEMS

There are many systemic health problems that either first manifest as a skin condition or have an associated skin change. It is nearly impossible to separate the integumentary status from other body systems, and the potential changes can be extensive. A few of the major skin changes that can occur with other health problems are as follows.

Identified Problem	Focused Question
Excessive sweating during the night	Have you been experiencing a cough or other respiratory health problem?
	Have you ever been tested for tuberculosis?
	Have you been losing weight for no apparent reason such as a diet change?
Itchy skin (appropriate for contact/allergic dermatitis or general pruritus)	How long has your skin been itchy?
	What helps the itchiness?

(*continued*)

(*continued*)

Identified Problem	Focused Question
	Where does the itchiness occur?
	Are there any red areas that are itchy or is the skin overall itchy?
	Have you changed the type of soap, laundry detergent, shampoo, lotion, perfume, or shaving cream lately?
	Is the itchiness more pronounced during a specific time of day?
	Does the itchiness prevent you from sleeping at night?
	What have you done to reduce the itching?
	Have you recently started taking any new medications?
	Have you talked with your (doctor, health care provider) about the itchiness?
	Have you ever been tested for allergies?
Draining wound	When did the wound first appear?
	Describe the size and color of the wound.
	Describe the drainage from the wound.
	What have you applied to the wound?
	What does the skin around the wound look like? Is it red or pale?
	What does the skin around the wound feel like? Is it cold or hot?
	Rate the amount of pain you are having from the wound on a scale of 1 to 10 with 1 being minimal or no pain to 10 being the worst possible pain.

(*continued*)

(*continued*)

Identified Problem	Focused Question
	Have you seen your doctor, health care professional about the wound?
	Does the wound appear to be healing or getting worse?
	Do you have a fever or other symptoms such as feeling tired or not having an appetite?
Foot wound	When did the foot wound first appear?
	How long have you had it?
	Describe the level of pain from the foot wound on a scale from 1 to 10 with 1 being minimal or no pain to 10 being the worst possible pain.
	What have you been doing to treat the foot wound?
	For what other health problems are you currently being treated?
	Have you seen your doctor or health care provider about the foot wound?
	What have you been instructed to do to treat the wound?
Edema	Do you have any areas of swelling around your ankles/feet/lower legs or hands?
	How long have you had these areas of swelling?
	Is the swelling always present?
	When did the swelling start?
	Does it get worse during the course of the day?
	Does elevating your (feet, legs, arms/hands) improve the swelling?

(*continued*)

(*continued*)

Identified Problem	Focused Question
	Does the swelling make it difficult to wear shoes?
	Do you need to take off your rings/ bracelets because of hand/arm swelling?
	When you press on the swollen area, is there an indentation made?
	How long does it take for the indentation to go away?
	When you experience this swelling, does your body weight also increase?
	Are you taking any medication for the swelling such as a diuretic?
	How long have you been taking this medication?
	What has your doctor or health care provider told you about the cause of the swelling?
	Is there anything specific that you are supposed to do when the swelling occurs?
Peripheral vascular disease	Is the color on your lower legs the same as the color on your upper legs?
	Is the color of your lower legs red/ brown in color?
	When did you first notice this change in color of your lower legs?
	Do your lower legs ache when you walk or do any other type of physical activity?
	Does the color of your lower legs change when the legs are elevated? Or when standing upright?

(*continued*)

(*continued*)

Identified Problem	Focused Question
	Does the skin over your lower legs appear shiny?
	Do you have hair growing over your lower legs? If not, when did the hair stop growing?
	Have you seen your doctor or health care provider about the changes in color, texture, or hair amount over your lower legs?
Cold hands/fingers	How long have you experienced cold hands/fingers?
	Do you smoke cigarettes?
	What is the color of the skin under your fingernails right now?
	Does the skin appear pink, red, or blue?
	Pinch one of your fingernails and then release the pinch. How long does it take for the color to return to the area?
	Have you seen your doctor or health care provider for your cold hands/fingers? What treatment has been prescribed?

ALGORITHM FOR THE INTEGUMENTARY SYSTEM

Finding	Action
Skin warm, dry, and intact	Move to assessing the hair
Skin dry and itchy	Assess medications. If new medications have been started, determine if adverse reactions include skin changes. If no new medications added, then assess fluid intake.

(*continued*)

(continued)

Finding	Action
	Fluid intake: If fluid intake has changed, assess for reasons. If no changes in fluid intake, then assess dietary intake.
	Dietary intake: Assess for routine dietary intake. If significant changes made to dietary intake, focus on changes which might impact skin status. If no changes in dietary intake, then assess alcohol intake.
	Alcohol intake: Assess for frequency and amount of alcohol intake. Determine if itchiness is associated with ingestion of alcohol. If no changes in alcohol intake, then assess urine output.
	Urine output: Assess frequency and estimated amount of urine output including frequency of voiding, color, presence of odor, etc.
Skin moist	Assess for recent infections. If no recent infection then assess for other causes to include changes in mentation, presence of a cough, or changes in body weight.
Skin breakdown/ wound	Assess when the wound occurred (any precipitating factors).
	Assess the length of time the wound has been present.
	What does the wound look like now? Describe the color of the wound bed.
	Describe the color and consistency of any wound drainage.
	Describe any odor that is associated with the wound.
	Estimate the size of the wound using household estimates such as the width of a finger, size of a quarter or other coin, width of an 8-ounce glass, etc.
	Describe any actions taken to treat the wound. What topical medication has been applied? Has the wound been covered with a bandage or left open to air?

(continued)

(continued)

Finding	Action
	Describe the condition of the skin around the wound. Is it red, swollen, painful, or pale and numb?
	Has the wound been seen by the doctor or health care provider? What treatment has been prescribed? Has the treatment improved the condition of the wound or made it worse?
Skin rash present	Assess location, appearance, characteristics to include color, shape, and if pruritus is present. Then assess for potential causes.
	Dietary intake: Assess for any alterations in usual diet. If no changes have occurred, assess for medications.
	Medications: Review all of the patient's current medications. Determine if any new ones have been added that correspond to the development of the rash. If medications have not been changed, assess environmental conditions.
	Environmental conditions: Have any changes been made to laundry detergent, bathing soap, shampoo, shaving cream, household cleaning products, or exposure to gardening pesticides. If no changes have occurred, assess for exposure to insects/vermin.
	Exposure to insects/vermin: Have you noticed or been exposed to spiders around or in your living environment? Have you noticed or been exposed to stinging insects such as bees/wasps/hornets? Have you noticed or been exposed to mosquitos? If no exposures proceed to assess for treatment options.
	Treatment options: Have you discussed the rash with your doctor or health care provider? What treatment has been prescribed? Has the treatment improved or made the condition worse?
Change in mole or skin tag	Determine the location of the mole/skin tag. Assess the previous appearance of the mole/skin tag and ask to describe how the mole/skin tag appears today. Include the following areas:

(continued)

(continued)

Finding	Action
	Color: What is the current color of the mole/skin tag?
	Condition: Is the mole/skin tag or the skin area around the mole/skin tag bleeding? When did you notice that the mole/skin tag had changed? Is the mole/skin tag tender/painful? If so, rate the pain on a scale from 1 to 10 with one being no or minimal pain and 10 being the worst pain possible.
	Actions: What have you done to treat the change in mole/skin tag? Have you discussed the mole/skin tag change with your doctor, health care provider?
Skin infection (folliculitis, carbuncle, furuncle)	Where is the skin infection located?
	How long has this infection been present?
	What does the skin area look like?
	Describe the condition of the skin around the infection.
	Describe any drainage coming out of the skin infection area.
	Rate the pain caused by the skin infection on a scale from 1 to 10 with one being minimal or no pain to 10 being the worst possible pain.
	Describe what has been done to treat the skin infection.
	Have you discussed the skin infection with your doctor, health care professional? What treatment has been prescribed? Has the treatment improved the skin infection or made it worse?

See Chapter 12 for additional information about integumentary system disorders.

TIPS WHEN ASSESSING THE INTEGUMENTARY SYSTEM

● Never diagnose a patient's skin condition. If the condition "sounds" serious or the patient expresses concern, strongly urge the patient to seek medical attention.

- Never recommend a medication or topical agent to be used on a skin condition. Ask the patient what has been used and document the skin's response to the treatment. If asked to recommend a treatment, strongly urge the patient to ask his or her doctor or health care provider.
- Do not minimize the skin condition. Avoid statements such as "that doesn't sound too bad," or "I'm sure that it's nothing." It is impossible to completely understand the type or extent of a skin condition or change without visualizing it. Encourage the patient to discuss the skin condition with his or her doctor or health care provider.

PRACTICE EXERCISES

1. A patient says that the skin of the lower legs has been warm with the recent development of small fluid-filled blisters.
   a. Which questions can be used to gain more information about the health problem?
2. A patient says that a mole on the left cheek has been getting progressively darker.
   a. What questions could be asked to learn more about this health problem?
   b. What guidance should you provide?
3. During the course of an assessment, the patient reports ingesting a six pack of beer and several ounces of whiskey every day.
   a. For which skin condition should you assess this patient?
4. A patient asks what "it means" when a skin wound is "black."
   a. What questions should be asked of this patient?
   b. What guidance should be strongly suggested to this patient?

CASE STUDY

Margaret Paul, an 80-year-old patient lives at home with her sister who is 75 years old. Margaret has been referred for telenursing care after being diagnosed with heart failure. She has a history of type 2 diabetes mellitus and has been using medication for glaucoma for several years. During the first telephone call, Margaret states that a wound has developed over the left lower leg, caused by bumping into the corner of an open dresser drawer in her bedroom.

- What questions would be a priority for Margaret?
- How does Margaret's history of type 2 diabetes mellitus impact the wound?
- What suggestions should you make to Margaret?

Margaret tells you that she is on Medicaid and has limited financial resources for medical care. Her sister wants to apply a homemade poultice of mustard and potatoes to place over the wound.

- What should you respond to the suggestion of a poultice?
- What other suggestions should you make considering Margaret's financial situation?

Margaret's sister gets on the telephone and begins to tell you that all health care providers are thieves and want to poison people with medications.

- How should you respond?
- What can you say to have Margaret continue to receive telephone calls in the future?

Margaret says that she needs to go, and you schedule a call in 5 days.

- What should you recommend to Margaret before ending the call?
- What else can you do to help this patient preserve her lower extremity?

KEY POINTS

- The integumentary system includes the skin, hair, and nails.
- This system is challenging to assess over the telephone because of the inability to visually see the skin.

- Use common household items to have the patient estimate the size of a skin rash, wound, or other lesion.
- Realize that a skin condition can be caused by a systemic illness.
- Never diagnose or suggest a treatment for a skin condition.

BIBLIOGRAPHY

Amirlak, B. (2015). Skin anatomy. *Medscape*. Retrieved from http://emedi cine.medscape.com/article/1294744-overview

D'Amico, D., & Barbarito, C. (2012). *Health and physical assessment in nursing* (2nd ed.). Upper Saddle River, NJ: Pearson.

Lemone, P. (2015). *Medical-surgical nursing* (6th ed.). Upper Saddle River, NJ: Pearson.

CHAPTER 6

Respiratory System

LEARNING OUTCOMES

Upon completion of this chapter, the nurse will:

1. Outline the areas to include when assessing the respiratory system
2. Identify appropriate questions to assess the respiratory system
3. Analyze approaches to gather more information about the respiratory system

THE RESPIRATORY SYSTEM

As a review, the respiratory system is divided into the upper and lower tracts. The parts of the upper respiratory tract include:

- Nose
- Sinuses
- Mouth
- Pharynx
- Larynx
- Part of the trachea

The major purpose of the upper respiratory tract is to moisten and warm inspired air. The sinuses:

- Decrease the weight of the skull bones
- Add resonance to the voice
- Protect delicate facial structures
- Produce mucus as part of the immune system

The pharynx is a part of both the respiratory and gastrointestinal systems. For the respiratory system, the pharynx:

- Moistens air
- Filters air

The main functions of the larynx are:

- Swallowing
- Talking
- Breathing

The trachea serves as a connection between the upper and lower respiratory tracts.

The lower respiratory tract consists of the connections from the trachea, the bronchi, and the lungs.

ASSESSMENT OVERVIEW

Because the respiratory system includes two sets of structures, the assessment should be divided into two parts. This assessment can be challenging. You will not be able to visualize:

- Nasal flaring
- Nasal drainage, color, and consistency
- Edematous sinus areas
- Chest drainage, color, and consistency
- Chest diameter
- Nail clubbing

Nurses traditionally use a stethoscope to listen for lung sounds. You will not be able to do this when providing telephonic care. What will be audible is the presence of a cough and the "noisiness" of breath sounds. The receiver on the telephone will serve as your "virtual" stethoscope. As with all major body system assessments, determine first if the patient is experiencing any particular respiratory problem. If so, focus on that area first. If not, complete a general assessment of this system.

QUESTIONS TO ASSESS THE RESPIRATORY SYSTEM

Upper Respiratory	
Component	**Question**
General	Have you noticed or experienced any changes in your breathing?
	If so, please describe the changes.
	How many pillows do you need or use to sleep and breathe comfortably?
	Has there been a change in the number of pillows you use?
	Have you ever been diagnosed with a respiratory problem?
	If so, what is the problem?
Nose	Do you breathe through your nose?
	Have you experienced any nasal stuffiness or congestion?
	Are you experiencing any nasal drainage?
	If so, what is the color of the drainage?
	Is there any particular pattern to your sneezing?
Mouth	Do you breathe through your mouth?
	If so, what is the primary reason for mouth-breathing?
Pharynx, larynx	Have you noticed any changes in your ability to swallow?
	Have you noticed any changes in your voice quality?
	If so, describe the changes.
Lower Respiratory	
Bronchi, lungs	Have you been experiencing a cough? (You will also be able to hear if the patient is coughing.)
	If so, how long have you had the cough?
	What causes the cough to occur?
	What make the cough better?
	Are you coughing up any phlegm?

(continued)

(*continued*)

Component	Question
	Describe the color of the phlegm.
	What does the cough sound like? ⊜ Dry? ⊜ Hacking/barking? ⊜ Moist/gurgling?
	Does the cough cause you any pain?
	If so, describe the pain: quality, location, intensity, and precipitating factors.
	Do you ever wake up from sleep coughing?
	If so, what do you do you to stop coughing?
General Concerns	
Environment	Do you have or have been diagnosed with allergies?
	To what are you allergic?
	Have you been prescribed medication to treat the allergies?
	How frequent do you experience respiratory effects from the allergies?
	Are you exposed to items in your work or home environment that affect your breathing or cause you to cough?
	Do you smoke?
	How much do you smoke? (Packs per day)
	When did you start smoking? (Pack years)
	Have you attempted smoking cessation?
	If so, when was the last time you stopped smoking?
	Do you use any other inhalants such as marijuana, vaping, glue, or spray paint?
	If so, how frequently do you use these inhalants?
Preventive measures	Do you receive an annual influenza vaccination?
	Have you ever received a vaccination for pneumonia? (appropriate for clients over the age of 65)

(*continued*)

(*continued*)

Component	Question
Physical changes	Have you noticed if your shirts or blouses are more snug across your chest?
	Have you noticed any changes in your fingernails? ● Are the tips of your fingers becoming thicker? ● Are the nails growing over the tips of the fingers? ● What is the color of your nail beds? Pink, pale, white-pale blue?

ASSESSING THE RESPIRATORY SYSTEM BY LISTENING

A great deal of information about the client's respiratory system can be collected by listening to the client talk/respond to questions. Assess for:

Shortness of breath	Can the client complete a sentence without having to stop and take a breath?
	Ask the client to walk to another part of the room. Listen to their ability to breath and talk while walking.
	After walking, ask if the client if he or she feels short of breath. You will be able to hear or determine this by the client's ability to talk, walk, or breathe.
	Does the client feel the need to sit down after walking a short distance?
Voice quality	Does the client's voice sound clear?
	Does the client sound "congested" or the voice has a "nasal" quality?
	Is the client "clearing the throat" while talking?
Lung sounds	Ask the client to take a deep breath in through the nose and exhale through the mouth. ● Are there any audible lung sounds? ● Wheezes? ● Rhonchi? ● Does the action of taking a deep breath in and out cause the client to cough?

ADDITIONAL ASSESSMENT QUESTIONS

Depending on the responses from the general assessment, you may want to collect additional data to determine if the client is experiencing a specific health problem. Questions to help with this data collection include the following:

Focused Questions	
New onset shortness of breath	Do you feel like you can't catch your breath?
	Has this ever happened before?
	What did you do to help it in the past?
	If this is new, suggest the client seek immediate medical attention.
Nose	Have you ever had a nosebleed?
	What did you do to control the bleeding?
	Are you experiencing that now? • If so, instruct to pinch the bridge of the nose and lean the head back against the back of a chair. • If the bleeding does not stop or slow down, suggest the client seek immediate medical attention.
Cough	What color is your phlegm?
	Have you coughed up this color of phlegm before?
	Is there blood in your phlegm? • If the client says the phlegm is dark in color or red, suggest that medical attention be sought immediately.
Throat	How long has your voice sounded hoarse or raspy?
	Has this ever happened to you before?
	What did you do to make the sound of your voice better?
	Are you experiencing any other symptoms like upper chest pain or swelling of the neck, face, or arms? • If pain or edema of the neck, face, or arms is present, suggest the client seek immediate medical attention.

ALGORITHM FOR ASSESSING THE RESPIRATORY SYSTEM

Finding	Action
Nasal stuffiness	Assess for other symptoms to include fever, cough, headache/sinus pressure
	Assess for self-treatment actions
	Suspect: allergies or a common cold
	Encourage to increase fluids
	Encourage to seek medical attention if symptoms persist
Cough	Assess for length of time cough has been occurring
	Assess for characteristics of sputum/phlegm production
	Assess for actions to self-treat the cough and effectiveness of actions
	Suspect: smoking history; chest cold/bronchitis; other lung infection
	Encourage to increase fluids
	Encourage to seek medical attention if cough persists
Shortness of breath	Assess for precipitating factors: activity, at rest, eating, while asleep
	Assess for length of time shortness of breath has been occurring
	Assess for actions taken to reduce episodes of shortness of breath
	Assess for associated symptoms such as nasal stuffiness or cough
	Assess if currently smoking cigarettes, exposed to cigarette smoking or other environmental irritants
	Suspect: chronic lung disease/infection; pneumonia; chronic heart condition
	Encourage to seek medical attention for ongoing shortness of breath

(continued)

(*continued*)

Finding	Action
Coughing blood	How long has this been going on?
	Are you having any chest pain?
	Describe the color: ● Dark red ● Light pink ● Streaks of blood
	What other health problems do you have?
	What medications are you taking? (assess for anticoagulants, aspirin)
	Suspect: infectious process (such as tuberculosis) or cancer pathology
	Encourage to seek medical attention for the bloody sputum

See Chapter 13 for additional information about respiratory system disorders.

PRACTICE EXERCISES

1. While conducting a wellness call the participant begins to cough.
   a. What characteristics of the cough should you document?
   b. What should you ask the participant about the cough?
2. Several times during a conversation the client stops talking and blows the nose.
   a. What questions should you ask about the nasal drainage?
3. During the course of a conversation about another health problem, the client asks "what does it mean when there's blood in my spit?"
   a. What questions would be a priority for you to ask?
   b. What should you encourage the patient to do?
4. While completing demographic information during the first call, the client needs to walk to another part of the room to locate the insurance card. You notice that, while he goes to the other part of the room, the client begins to pant/breathe faster and is unable to verbally complete a sentence while walking.

a. What should you focus on during the next few questions?
b. What health problems should you suspect this client might be experiencing?

CASE STUDY

Situation 1

Marilyn works for an insurance company as a telephonic nurse and is scheduled to contact a newly enrolled member for a wellness call. After identifying the purpose of the call and validating the member's identity, Marilyn notices that the client has a nasal quality to the voice and periodically clears the throat while talking.

- What should Marilyn suspect the member is experiencing?
- What questions would be appropriate for Marilyn to ask the member at this time?
  The member states that during the spring and fall, nasal stuffiness and congestion occurs almost daily. At times the throat becomes very dry, and thick mucus causes the voice to sound harsh.
- What additional questions should Marilyn ask?
- What information would be used to differentiate seasonal allergies from a more severe health problem?

Situation 2

Larry is a telephonic nurse working for an agency that provides wellness calls. Currently, Larry is preparing to contact an employee of a manufacturing plant.
  The employee is not eager to talk; however, the employee agrees to spend a few minutes. During the first few sentences, Larry realizes that the employee is short of breath and seems to pause and breathe before talking or completing a sentence.

- Why should Larry include an assessment of the respiratory system during the call?
- For what environmental conditions should Larry assess?

- What should Larry do if the employee is exposed to sawdust and aerated chemicals while on the job?
- What information should Larry share once learning that the employee has smoked one ppd for 17 years?

TIPS FOR ASSESSING THE RESPIRATORY SYSTEM

- Be sure that you are in a quiet environment.
- Take your time and listen closely to the client's voice and breathing pattern.
- Stop and listen if the client begins to cough or is coughing. Consider the characteristics of the cough and possible causes.
- Have the client be your "eyes." Ask if upper body clothing isn't "fitting" the same. This could indicate a change in A-P (anterior–posterior chest) diameter seen in people who are barrel-chested because of chronic lung problems. Ask if there have been any changes in the finger nails/tips of the fingers. Are the fingers becoming wider and the nails growing over the edges? This helps determine if the client has clubbing.
- For any clients who currently smoke cigarettes, gently offer information about smoking cessation. Accept the client's response. Do not push for smoking cessation if it is not desired or welcomed by the client.

KEY POINTS

- Not every client will need a complete or focused respiratory assessment.
- Ask if the client is experiencing any breathing problems at this time. If not, then there is no need to conduct a full assessment.
- Be aware of the client's ability to respond to questions. If shortness of breath is present, keep the call short and increase the frequency of the calls in the future.
- Do not assume that every client with nasal congestion or cough has a chronic condition.
- Remember to not diagnose any health problem. If the client is concerned about any symptom, strongly suggest the client discuss the issue with a doctor or health care provider.

BIBLIOGRAPHY

D'Amico, D., & Barbarito, C. (2012). *Health and physical assessment in nursing* (2nd ed.). Upper Saddle River, NJ: Pearson.

Lemone, P. (2015). *Medical–surgical nursing* (6th ed.). Upper Saddle River, NJ: Pearson.

CHAPTER 7

Cardiovascular System

LEARNING OUTCOMES

Upon completion of this chapter, the nurse will:

1. Outline the areas to include when assessing the cardiovascular system
2. Identify appropriate questions to assess the cardiovascular system
3. Analyze approaches to gather more information about the cardiovascular system

THE CARDIOVASCULAR SYSTEM

The cardiovascular system includes the heart, blood vessels, lymphatic system, and components of the blood. Before focusing on the assessment of this system, a brief review of each component might be helpful.

The Heart

As a review, the heart:

- Is a "double pump"
- Is composed of three layers of thick muscle
- Has four chambers: two atria and two ventricles
- Has an independent conduction system that stimulates contraction
- Has four valves that create heart sounds
- Is nourished through the coronary arteries
- Plays an active role in blood pressure regulation
- Is affected by electrolyte and fluid balance

Arterial Circulation

The arteries carry oxygenated blood to all body organs and tissues. This structure is composed of three layers of tissue—tunica intima, media, and adventitia—which play a role in blood pressure regulation. The pumping action of the heart in addition to blood viscosity and vessel wall integrity influence arterial circulation. The integrity of the peripheral arterial system is evaluated when assessing peripheral pulses in the arm/hand, neck, groin, knee, ankle, and foot.

Venous Circulation

The veins carry deoxygenated blood. These vessels are thicker and rely on muscular contraction, pressure changes with breathing, and one-way valves to ensure blood return back to the heart.

Lymphatic System

This system plays a role in infection control and total body immunity. It consists of a network of vessels that drain into two major lymphatic ducts located on each side of the body. Lymph nodes are located throughout the body and collect fluid and other debris.

The Blood

The blood is made up of red and white blood cells and plasma. The blood has many purposes, to include:

- Transporting oxygen to body tissues
- Removing carbon dioxide and other body wastes
- Fighting infection
- Transporting electrolytes and fluids to maintain balance

Hemoglobin measures the oxygen-carrying capacity of the red blood cells. Hematocrit is the percentage of red blood cells within the entire circulation.

ASSESSMENT OVERVIEW

Because the cardiovascular system has several different parts, it makes sense to focus on one section at a time. As a telephonic nurse you will be limited in your ability to:

- Visualize skin color
- Perform capillary filling time
- Palpate peripheral pulses
- Auscultate heart sounds
- Visualize the skin for bruising
- Palpate lower extremities for peripheral edema
- Palpate lymph nodes
- Measure blood pressure

However, when conducting a telephonic assessment of this system you will use careful questioning to gather important information. Keep in mind that the cardiovascular and respiratory systems are intimately related. Because of this, some of the assessment questions may be appropriate for either body system. As with all major body system assessments, determine first if the patient is experiencing any particular cardiovascular problem. If so, focus on that area first. If not, complete a general assessment of this system.

QUESTIONS TO ASSESS THE CARDIOVASCULAR SYSTEM

Structure/ System	Question
Heart	How would you rate your energy level? Good, fair, poor?
	Have you ever been told that you have a heart problem?
	Have you ever had an electrocardiogram (EKG)?
	Have you ever been told that you have an irregular heart rhythm?
	Do you ever feel like your heart skips a beat or "changes gears"?
	Do you ever feel like your heart is beating fast?
	Do you ever feel like there is a bird fluttering in your chest?

(continued)

(continued)

Structure/ System	Question
	Have you ever passed out (lost consciousness) without any known reason?
	Have you ever had an infection that affected your heart?
	Have you ever had surgery on your heart as an adult or as a child?
	Have you ever experienced chest pain? • If so, described the pain.
	Describe the color of the skin under your fingernails. Would you say that it is: pink, red, white, pale?
	Listen to the client talk and if a cough is present. If coughing, note if it sounds dry or moist. If it sounds moist ask: • How long have you had a cough? • Do you produce any phlegm? • Does the phlegm appear pink in color?
Arterial circulation	Have you ever been told that you have a problem with any of your arteries? If so, which ones?
	When was the last time that you had your blood pressure measured? • If so, do you remember what the numbers were?
	Do you ever wake up with a headache?
	Do you ever experience blurred vision?
	Do you ever have nosebleeds? • If so, when was the last nosebleed? • How long did it last? • What did you do to make it stop?
	Have you been prescribed or are taking medication for high blood pressure? If so: • What is the name of your medication? • How often do you take it? • How long have you been taking it? • Have you had any problems or side effects from taking this medication?
	Is the color of your lower legs the same color as the rest of your skin?

(continued)

(*continued*)

Structure/ System	Question
	Do you have any swelling around your feet or ankles?
	Do you have any numbness or tingling of your feet or hands?
	Do you ever have pain in your calves (the back of your lower legs) when you walk? If so: ⦿ How would you describe the pain? (The pain of arterial insufficiency is often described as sharp or stabbing.) ⦿ Does exercise or walking make it better or worse? (Walking will make arterial insufficiency worse.) ⦿ How long does it last? ⦿ What do you do to make it stop? ⦿ Does elevating your legs make the pain better or worse?
	Have you noticed if the amount of hair on your lower legs has changed?
	Does the skin of your lower legs appear shiny?
	Do you smoke cigarettes or use any tobacco products? ⦿ If so, for how long? (pack years) ⦿ How much do you smoke or use tobacco products?
Venous circulation	Is the skin over the front of your lower legs darker in color than the rest of the skin on your legs?
	Do you have any wounds or sores on your legs or ankles? If so: ⦿ How long have you had these sores? ⦿ What have you been using to treat the sores?
	Do you ever experience swelling of your legs and ankles? ⦿ If so, does elevating your legs make the swelling go down?
	Do your legs swell if you sit or stand in one position too long?
	How would you rate your activity level? ⦿ Active (participate in sports or other activity daily) ⦿ Moderate (participate in sports or other activity a few times a week) ⦿ Sedentary (limited to household chores)

(*continued*)

(continued)

Structure/ System	Question
	Do you ever experience pain in your lower legs? If so: ● Describe the pain. (The pain of venous insufficiency is often described as a feeling of fullness or aching.) ● Does walking make the pain better or worse? ● How long does the pain last? ● What do you do to make the pain stop or improve?
	Have you ever been diagnosed with varicose veins? If so: ● What treatment have you received, if any? ● What do you do to reduce the discomfort from the varicose veins?
Lymphatic system	Do you have any swellings? ● On your neck? ● Around your upper chest/armpits? ● One arm or hand? ● Groin? ● One leg?
	Have you ever been told or diagnosed with a problem with your lymph system or drainage?
	Have you had any surgeries that interrupt lymph drainage such as surgery for breast cancer?
	Do you ever get "swollen glands" with an infection or chest cold?
	Have you ever had to be hospitalized for the infection and the swollen glands?
	Have you ever been diagnosed or treated for cancer that affects the lymph or glands?
Blood	Have you ever been told or diagnosed with a problem with your blood? If so, please describe the problem.
	Have you ever been diagnosed with anemia caused by low iron?
	Have you ever been diagnosed with anemia caused by something else?

(continued)

(*continued*)

Structure/ System	Question
	Do you take or have been prescribed medication to treat anemia? If so: ⚬ What is the name of the medication? ⚬ How long have you been taking it? ⚬ How many times a day do you take it? ⚬ Is it a pill or do you have to get injections?
	Do you ever get short of breath when you do routine activities? (This question might be inappropriate if the client smokes. If the client does not smoke, shortness of breath can be an indication of a low hemoglobin level.)
	Do you take or have been prescribed any medication that makes your blood thinner? If so: ⚬ What is the name of the medication? ⚬ How long have you been taking the medication? ⚬ How many times a day do you take it?
	Do you ever get any bruises on your skin that just occur without any injury? ⚬ Where are these bruises located? ⚬ How long do they last? ⚬ Do they routinely reappear?
	Do your gums bleed easily when brushing your teeth? ⚬ How long has this been going on? ⚬ Have you discussed this with your doctor, dentist, health care provider?
	When you get a minor cut or scrape of the skin, how long does it take for the area to stop bleeding? ⚬ Do you have to apply pressure to the area to make it stop bleeding?
	Have you ever been told or diagnosed with a health problem that affects your blood's ability to clot such as hemophilia? If so: ⚬ Do you know the type of hemophilia? ⚬ Have you had to be hospitalized for treatment of the hemophilia? ⚬ Do you take medication for the hemophilia?

(*continued*)

(*continued*)

Structure/ System	Question
	Do you recall the last time that you had an infection? If so: • What type of infection was it? • Were you prescribed antibiotics for the infection? • Has the infection reappeared since the last treatment?
	How often do you experience a fever? If frequently: • Is there a particular time of day when the fever occurs? • What do you do to treat the fever? • Do you experience extreme sweating when the fever breaks?
	Do you take or have been prescribed a medication called a steroid? If so: • Why were you prescribed this medication? • Are you still taking this medication? • Can you recall the last time you had to take this medication? • How long did you take it?

ALGORITHM FOR ASSESSING THE CARDIOVASCULAR SYSTEM

As you can see, the assessment of the cardiovascular system can be lengthy. You might want to change your approach when assessing this system to focus on specific problematic areas. Suggestions to streamline the assessment are as follows:

Finding	Action
Chest pain	Assess the pain for: • Quality • Location • Radiation to the arm or jaw area • Associated with nausea/vomiting • Sweating
	Assess how long it has been going on
	Suspect an acute myocardial infarction if this is a new episode and direct to seek immediate medical attention

(*continued*)

(*continued*)

Finding	Action
	Suspect angina if this has happened before ● Assess if client has medication to treat the chest pain ● Suggest the client follow the directions to treat the chest pain
Dysrhythmia	Assess if the client has a history of an irregular heartbeat
	Assess if the client ever feels like the heart is skipping beats
	Assess if prescribed medication to treat the irregular heartbeat
	Suspect a ventricular dysrhythmia (premature ventricular contractions)
	Assess if the client is experiencing palpitations or fluttering. If so, determine: ● Frequency ● Time the discomfort has been occurring
	Any associated factors such as: ● Occurs after ingesting something containing caffeine (coffee) or chocolate ● Occurs during or after smoking
	Suspect an atrial dysrhythmia (premature atrial contractions, atrial fibrillation, atrial flutter)
	Encourage to seek medical attention
Heart failure	Assess if the client has a history of foot/ankle/lower leg swelling
	Assess if the client has a cough. Determine if the cough "sounds" productive. If so, ask: ● How long has the cough been occurring? ● Is there any phlegm produced? ● The color of the phlegm?
	Assess if the client has noticed the veins in the neck being more prominent than usual
	Assess if the client has ever been told or diagnosed with "heart failure"

(*continued*)

(continued)

Finding	Action
	Assess if the client takes or is prescribed medications for the "heart failure." If so, ● What is the name of the medication? ● How long has the medication been prescribed? ● How many times a day is the medication taken?
	Assess if the client is experiencing any new symptoms of the "heart failure"
	Encourage the client to discuss the new symptoms with the doctor or health care provider
Problems with circulation	Assess if there is a change in the color of the skin over the lower extremities
	Assess if the feet and legs feel cold or warm to touch
	Assess if the feet/legs feel numb
	Assess if the skin appears shiny or if there is a change in the amount of body hair over the lower extremities
	Assess if there is any swelling of the feet/ankles/lower legs
	Assess if there are any wounds on the legs
	Assess if the client is experiencing any pain with activity and inactivity
	Suspect arterial insufficiency if the skin is red in color and experiences pain with walking or other activity.
	Suspect venous insufficiency if the skin is dark brown and experiencing a feeling of heaviness or fullness of the legs when sitting or standing in the same position
	Encourage discussing the issues with circulation with the doctor or health care provider
Swollen glands	Assess the location of the swollen gland (the neck, under the arm, in the groin)
	Assess how long the gland has been swollen
	Assess if the swollen gland is painful to touch
	Assess if the swollen gland can move or is fixed or feels like it is sticking to one area

(continued)

(*continued*)

Finding	Action
	Assess if the swollen gland feels like rubber or harder like a marble
	Suspect an acute infection if the swollen gland is movable and rubbery
	Suspect another disease process if the swollen gland is hard and immovable
	Encourage discussing the swollen gland with the doctor or health care provider
New onset of morning headache, blurred vision, and nosebleed	Assess where the headache is located? • Around the back of the neck • Throughout the forehead
	Assess if the headache gets better as the day progresses?
	Assess what has been done for the headache: • Taking over-the-counter medication • Laying down with a cool compress
	Assess when the blurred vision first started
	Assess if the client participates in any activities that could cause eyestrain: needlepoint, reading small print, extensive computer work, etc.
	Assess if there are any other eye changes noticed: tearing, crusting, redness, drainage
	Assess what the client was doing when the nosebleed started
	Assess how long the bleed lasted
	Assess what was done, if anything, to help stop the bleeding
	Suspect an elevation in blood pressure
	Encourage to see the doctor or health care provider for the new symptoms and to have blood pressure measured as soon as possible
New onset of fatigue	Assess how long the fatigue has been occurring
	Assess when the fatigue was first noticed

(*continued*)

(*continued*)

Finding	Action
	Assess what is being done about the fatigue
	Assess if the fatigue is associated with anything else such as: • New onset of productive cough • New onset of foot/ankle/lower extremity swelling • Change in amount of urine output • Change in appetite • Blurred vision • Headache • Irritability • Shortness of breath or difficulty "catching the breath" • New onset of numbness or tingling of the feet/hands • Inability to complete activities of daily living without having to stop and rest
	Suspect exacerbation or new onset of heart failure if fatigue is associated with productive cough, lower extremity edema, change in urine output, change in appetite, shortness of breath, irritability
	Suspect acute elevation of blood pressure if fatigue is associated with blurred vision and headache
	Suspect anemia for the fatigue is associated with shortness of breath, activity intolerance, or numbness/tingling of the hands/feet
	Encourage to talk with the doctor or health care provider about the symptoms
Unexplained bruising	Assess where the bruises are located
	Assess for the estimated size of the bruises
	Assess if the bruises are "clustered" around a joint such as the knee or ankle or scattered over a large area such as over both arms, both legs, the abdomen, the lower back, etc.
	Assess if the client recalls bumping into anything (furniture, car door) that could have caused the bruising
	Assess if the bruises are painful
	Assess if experiencing any new onset of bleeding gums, nosebleed, or coughing of blood

(*continued*)

(continued)

Finding	Action
	Suspect an alteration in platelets/clotting with a new unexplained onset of bruising
	Encourage to discuss the bruising with the doctor or health care provider
Experiencing fevers	Assess when the fevers were first noticed
	Assess if the fevers occur during any particular time of day
	Assess if the fevers are associated with any other symptoms or body changes
	Assess what the client has been doing to treat the fevers
	Assess if the fevers are occurring more or less frequently
	Encourage to discuss the new onset of fevers with the doctor or health care provider
New onset of swollen feet, ankles, or legs	Assess the area that is edematous
	Assess if the client can see an indentation when the swollen area is pressed with a finger
	Assess when client measured body weight
	Assess if the weight has increased since the last measurement
	Assess if there has been a change in amount of urine voided
	Assess if the client has increased the amount of salt ingested
	Assess if the client has noticed tightness or swelling of the fingers/hands and/or under/around the eyes
	Suspect acute fluid volume overload (which can be due to heart failure, renal failure, hypertension)
	Encourage to discuss the new onset of swelling with the doctor or health care provider

See Chapter 14 for additional information about cardiovascular system disorders.

TIPS FOR ASSESSING THE CARDIOVASCULAR SYSTEM

- Clients may not understand the term dysrhythmia or arrhythmia. Asking about having an irregular heartbeat may provide more information for you.
- Clients may not consider swelling of the feet or ankles as being unusual. Ask if the client notices that the shoes feel tight at the end of the day. You could also ask if the client's rings are fitting tighter on the fingers. Some clients may be dismayed about a new onset of "gaining weight in the belly." This could be ascites or sacral edema. Carefully assess how long this has been going on, if there has been an associated weight gain, and if the doctor or health care provider has been contacted about it.
- Clients may react negatively to the term "heart failure." Consider asking if the client has ever been told that they have extra "fluid in their heart or lungs" or have to take a "water pill" to get rid of extra body water.
- Stay calm when discussing symptoms that the client may be experiencing. The client may already be anxious about a symptom and could be seeking reassurance from you during the call. Do not make any rote comments such as "I'm sure that is nothing" or "don't worry about it." Encourage the client to see the doctor or health care provider for additional evaluation.
- Be aware of the client's energy level while on the call. If the client is short of breath you will need to keep the call short and schedule follow-up calls more frequently.
- Focus on the symptom and if the client has any other health problems that could be causing the symptom. Shortness of breath can be caused by a lung problem, heart problem, or anemia. Avoid assuming that the symptom is an extension of another problem but rather ascertain if it is new.
- Be aware of your organization's approach to emergency situations. Do not automatically direct clients to call an ambulance for emergency assistance unless it is truly an emergency and you fear that the client could lose consciousness while on the telephone. Not all clients have an ambulance benefit with their health plans and calling for emergency services that were not truly necessary could cause the client financial hardship. Always ask if the client's doctor or health care provider is aware of the symptom before directing the client to seek immediate medical attention.

- Do not automatically assume that bruising is caused by a bleeding disorder. Some medications have bruising as an adverse effect. Review the client's current medications first and determine if any could be causing the bruising.
- Remember that not all clients will willingly discuss health problems. You may find the client answering questions briskly, ending the call abruptly, or changing the topic. Should this occur, ask if the client is experiencing any new problems and wants to talk about them now.

PRACTICE EXERCISES

Read the following client situations and determine:

- Which questions to ask
- What the client might be experiencing
- Whether the situation is an emergency

1. A client who is newly enrolled in a health plan is added to the call list because of recent blood work for electrolytes and a lipid panel. During the call the client has a productive cough and occasionally incorrectly answers questions.
2. An employee is added to a wellness program. During the call the employee mentions occasional nosebleeds after participating in sporting activities associated with a headache across the forehead. The bleeding stops after a few minutes and doesn't occur with any other activities.
3. A client mentions that the left foot and ankle have been swelling occasionally. The entire left lower leg feels heavier than the right but has no other pain. The skin over the lower leg is not shiny and has no change in hair distribution or amount. The color is slightly more red than the right leg but does not feel warm to touch. Overnight the swelling of the left foot and lower leg goes away but returns depending on how much time the client has to sit at work.
4. A client newly enrolled in a disease management program has shortness of breath and cannot complete a full sentence without having to stop and take a breath. The client takes heart medication and a "water pill" but feels "bloated" and hasn't been "passing water" as much as usual.

5. A client calls into the organization asking to speak to a nurse because of sudden severe chest pain. The pain does not radiate down the arm or up the neck but feels like sharp stabs that occur periodically in a rhythm. The pain does not change when taking a deep breath and is not associated with nausea, vomiting, sweating, or feeling like the heart is pounding.

6. During a routine call, a client newly enrolled in a health plan asks if it means anything if there are new bruises around both ankles.

7. A client in a disease management program says that even after getting 9 hours of sleep he still feels tired and unable to shower, dress, make the bed, or get something to eat. This is the first time that he has felt this "bad" and has an appointment scheduled with the doctor in 2 weeks

8. During a follow-up call a client begins to experience chest pain. The client says that she's had this before but never while sitting down or talking on the telephone.

9. A client denies having any history of heart or circulation problems. During the assessment, the client states that occasionally the heart pounds, especially after drinking a large cup of coffee, and at times it feels like the heart is speeding up and then slowing down. The client does not feel faint or have any other symptoms.

10. During the course of a call, a client asks why a headache would occur every morning but goes away in a few hours.

CASE STUDY

Kacey is scheduled to call a member newly enrolled in a disease management program. During the initial call, Kacey notes that the client makes "gurgling" sounds when breathing and talking. The client admits to having a "heart problem" but does not know the official term. Even when denying shortness of breath, Kacey notes that the client stops talking to take a breath. During the medication review, Kacey learns that the client takes a "water pill" and two "heart pills." The client mentions having a doctor's appointment the next day and agrees to call Kacey afterwards to report the results of the examination.

- What health problem do you think the client is experiencing?
- What other information would be helpful to have about this client's symptoms?

Kacey notes that the client does not call into the office the next day and decides to give the client a call. The telephone is not answered, and Kacey leaves a message, asking the client to return the call whenever convenient.

- Where might the client be?
- What findings from the previous call might have indicated that the client was experiencing an acute exacerbation of a chronic illness?

Several weeks pass, and Kacey takes an inbound call. It is the client who has been missing! Kacey learns that when the client went to the doctor's office, an ambulance was called, and the client was admitted to the hospital for "fluid in the lungs." The client had a "breathing tube" for about a week and then had to go to "rehab" to "get my strength back." The client is going to have physical therapy in the home three times a week and has a follow-up appointment with the doctor in a month.

- What is important to ask the client at this time?
- Should a review of medications occur again?
- Why do you think the client is getting physical therapy in the home?

Kacey notes that the client is able to talk in full sentences and no longer hears "gurgling" on the phone. The client admits to feeling occasionally fatigued but gets more energy after resting for about 30 minutes a "couple of times" a day.

- Should you be concerned about the client's fatigue?
- What should you do to make sure that this client is not rehospitalized for the same problem?
- How frequent do you think this client should be contacted?
- What additional information from the first call might have been helpful to have to reduce this client's risk of needing to be hospitalized?

KEY POINTS

- The cardiovascular system includes the heart, arterial and venous blood vessels, the lymphatic system, and the blood.

- Begin the assessment by asking if the client has been experiencing any particular problems with the system. If there are no particular problems, a general review of each of the major areas can be completed.
- If a client is experiencing a new problem within the cardiovascular system, carefully assess the symptoms and encourage the client to see the doctor/health care provider.
- If the client has a known cardiac problem, refer to a later chapter for more specific information about assessment approaches.
- Remember that there is no one "right way" to complete a cardiovascular assessment. Follow the client's lead. You might find yourself "jumping around" during the call. This is perfectly acceptable and communicates that you are doing more than "collecting information" from the client.
- Be aware of breathing difficulties or fatigue during a call.
- Find out if the client has an ambulance benefit before suggesting emergency medical care.

BIBLIOGRAPHY

D'Amico, D., & Barbarito, C. (2012). *Health and physical assessment in nursing* (2nd ed.). Upper Saddle River, NJ: Pearson.

Innerbody.com. (2016). Cross-section of artery and vein. Retrieved from http://www.innerbody.com/image/card05.html

Lemone, P. (2015). *Medical–surgical nursing* (6th ed.). Upper Saddle River, NJ: Pearson.

Pearson Education. (2015). *Nursing: A concept-based approach to learning* (2nd ed., Vol. 2). Upper Saddle River, NJ: Author.

CHAPTER 8

Gastrointestinal System

LEARNING OUTCOMES

Upon completion of this chapter, the nurse will:

1. Outline the areas to include when assessing the gastrointestinal system
2. Identify appropriate questions to assess the gastrointestinal system
3. Analyze approaches to gather more information about the gastrointestinal system

THE GASTROINTESTINAL SYSTEM

The primary function of the gastrointestinal system is digestion. The organs and structures within the system are extensive and include:

- Mouth
- Esophagus
- Stomach
- Small intestine
  - Duodenum
  - Jejunum
  - Ileum
- Large intestine
  - Cecum
  - Ascending colon
  - Transverse colon
  - Descending colon
  - Sigmoid colon
  - Rectum
  - Anus

The organs of digestion need assistance for food to be absorbed and utilized by the body. These accessory organs include:

- Liver
- Gallbladder
- Pancreas

As a review, after swallowing food that is chewed in the mouth, it travels through the esophagus to the stomach where it begins to be broken down and converted into a substance called chyme. Once chyme enters the small intestine, it is further broken down by enzymes secreted by the liver, gallbladder, and pancreas in preparation for being absorbed. Once all potential substances are absorbed, the residue from the food is advanced to the beginning of the large intestine where any additional water from the food residue is absorbed. At the completion of this entire process, the remnants of ingested food are eliminated in the stool.

Although this process sounds easy, many things impact a well-functioning gastrointestinal system. First of all, a person needs to have an appetite in order to seek food. Then, adequate dentition and sufficient saliva are needed to wet the food and begin the breaking down process. The esophagus needs to be intact with a functioning cardiac sphincter to prevent food from backing up from the stomach. The stomach needs to have sufficient hydrochloric acid to prepare chyme and an intact pyloric sphincter to prevent reflux of chyme once it advances into the small intestine. The liver, gallbladder, and pancreas need to be functioning at a high level in order to break down proteins, carbohydrates, and fats for body absorption. And the large intestine needs to be clear and free of inflammation in order to adequately remove food residue from the body.

ASSESSMENT OVERVIEW

Because the gastrointestinal system involves many parts and body organs, it is best to approach the assessment methodically. As with other body organs, the traditional methods to assess this system telephonically are different. You will need to focus on thoughtful questioning and careful listening when completing the assessment of this body system.

Keep in mind that you will not be able to:

- Inspect the condition of the oral cavity including dentition
- Auscultate bowel sounds
- Palpate the abdomen
- Percuss the abdomen
- Observe the color of emesis or stool
- Test stool for occult blood
- Further assess stool for steatorrhea
- Observe skin color for jaundice

Because the organs within this system are grouped as primary and accessory, assessment can occur following the same approach. Remember that most people do not like to spend time discussing their digestion and bowel function. For some, this can be uncomfortable, and a patient/client may provide short answers without divulging what they consider intimate information. A "matter of fact" conversational approach is recommended to gather the most quality information.

QUESTIONS TO ASSESS THE GASTROINTESTINAL SYSTEM

As with other system assessments, begin by asking if the patient has had any problems with eating or digesting food. If the answer is "no," you can conduct a general assessment of all major gastrointestinal organs. You can begin the assessment of this system by introducing the questioning with a general statement such as:

- "I'm glad to hear that you don't have any issues with eating or digestion. Let's just take a few minutes anyway and go over some specific areas."

Some seasoned telephonic nurses like to begin the assessment of the gastrointestinal system by asking the patient for his or her height and current weight. From this information, the nurse then proceeds into the general questions. This approach is appropriate for some patients but not for others. Use your best judgment. There is no "right or wrong" time to gather height/weight information.

Structure	Question
Mouth	Do you have any problems chewing food?
	Do you have all or most of your teeth? If not, do you have: • A partial plate? • Dentures? If dentures, are they: • Well fitting? • Are you experiencing any sores or bleeding of your gums from the dentures?
	Do you have any problems with swallowing fluid or food? If so, do you: • Cough when you swallow food or fluid?
Esophagus	Does it ever feel like food gets "stuck" in your throat after swallowing? If so, • What do you do to help this? ▪ Eat more food? ▪ Drink some fluid? ▪ Burp?
Stomach	Have you ever been diagnosed or told that you have a stomach problem?
	Do you ever experience pain or burning from your stomach? If so, • Does the pain/burning occur before eating? • During eating? • If it occurs after eating, how long after eating does the pain occur?
	Do you take any medicine for your stomach? Is it for: • Absorption? (enzymes) • Digestion? (enzymes) • Vitamin supplement? (Vitamin B_{12}, iron) • Indigestion? (chewable tablets)
	Have you noticed any change in your appetite? Describe the change such as: • No desire to eat • Desire to eat only one type of food • Appetite has been increasing with no associated weight gain • Weight gain despite not ingesting a routine amount of food
	How long is it between meals before you start to feel hungry again?

(continued)

(continued)

Structure	Question
	When you feel hungry do you seek food to eat or do you ignore the hunger and eat later? ● How long do you wait after hunger pains to eat? ● How many meals do you eat a day? ● How many snacks do you eat a day?
	Does nausea ever prevent you from eating? If so, ● How often would you say you are nauseated? ● Do you ever vomit after feeling nauseated? ● How often does this occur?
	Are there any foods that cause you to become immediately ill? If so, ● What are the foods? ● Have you been told you have food allergies? ● What happens if you eat a food that you are allergic to? ● What do you do if you accidentally eat a food that you are allergic to?
	Have you ever had testing done for your stomach such as ● Swallow barium? ● Scope of your stomach to look at the lining?
Small intestine	Do you ever experience a burning sensation around your belly button? If so, ● What do you do when this happens? ● Have you talked with your doctor or health care provider about it?
	Do you ever hear your stomach gurgling? If so, ● Do you hear it a lot? ● When does it most often occur? ● Does anything else happen when the gurgling occurs such an episode of diarrhea or the need to have a regular bowel movement?
	Do you ever feel like your abdomen or belly is swollen or bloated? If so, ● How often does this occur? ● What makes it better? ● Do you take any medicine for the bloating? ● Have you talked about this with your doctor or health care provider?

(continued)

(*continued*)

Structure	Question
	Have you ever had testing done on your small intestine such as: ● Swallow barium?
Large intestine	Are you currently experiencing any problems with your bowels?
	How often do you have a bowel movement? ● What is considered a normal bowel movement frequency for you?
	Describe the color and shape of your routine bowel movement.
	Does the shape of your bowel movement ever change, such as: ● Thin like a pencil? ● Small hard round pieces?
	Does your bowel movement ever seem: ● Lighter in color than usual? ● Darker in color than usual?
	Does your bowel movement ever have particles of undigested food in it?
	Do you have any problems with having a routine bowel movement? If so, ● Is the stool hard and difficult to pass? ● Is the stool runny? ● Does the stool have a strong or odor that is unusual for you? ● Do you ever have obvious blood in or around your stool? ● Does your stool ever look black and sticky like tar?
	Do you ever experience diarrhea? If so, ● How often? ● Does anything make it happen? ● Do you have any pain with it? ● Do you take anything over-the-counter to make it stop? ● Have you talked with your doctor or health care provider about it? ● Have you been prescribed medicine to make it stop?

(*continued*)

(continued)

Structure	Question
	Do you take anything to help with bowel movements? If so, ◦ What do you take? ◦ How often do you take it? ◦ How long have you been taking it? ◦ Have you discussed the need to take something to have a bowel movement with your doctor or health care provider?
	Have you had any testing done on your bowels such as: ◦ Have an enema using barium
	Have you ever had a colonoscopy? If so, ◦ When was it done? ◦ What was the outcome? ◦ Did your doctor or health care provider prescribe anything after your colonoscopy?
Rectum/ anus	Have you ever been told you have hemorrhoids? If so, ◦ What has been prescribed to treat them? ◦ How often do they "bother" you? ◦ Do you take any over-the-counter preparations for them? ◦ Does your doctor or health care provider suggest that you have surgery to remove them? If so, ▪ When was it done/when will it be done?
Liver	Have you ever been diagnosed or told that you have a problem with your liver? If so, ◦ What have you been told? ◦ How long have you been having problems with your liver? ◦ Do you take any medicine for your liver problem? ◦ Do you need to avoid anything because of your liver such as: ▪ Tylenol? ▪ Alcohol? ◦ Did your skin ever have a yellow color? If so, ▪ Is it yellow now? ◦ If it was yellow in the past, how long did it last? ◦ Did it ever turn yellow again?

(continued)

(*continued*)

Structure	Question
	Have you been told to avoid any foods because of your liver?
	Have you ever been in the hospital because of a liver problem? If so, • Did you ever have to have fluid taken out of your belly because of your liver? • Did you ever have to have a tube in your nose because of bleeding caused by your liver?
Gall-bladder	Have you ever been told that you have a problem with your gallbladder? If so, • Were you told that you have stones?
	Have you ever had bowel movements that looked like they didn't have any color/were not brown? If so, • How long did that last? • What was done about it?
	Do you ever have any pain that you have been told is caused by your gallbladder?

	If you have had pain, was the pain:
	• Around your right shoulder blade on your back?
	• How long does the pain last?
	• What do you do for the pain? Do you:
	  ▪ Take over-the-counter medicine?
	  ▪ Avoid eating a certain type of food?

	Have you had/are going to have surgery to remove your gallbladder? • When was/will it be done? • Are you experiencing any other problems after having your gallbladder removed?
Pancreas	Have you ever been told that you have a problem with your pancreas? If so, what is it?
	Have you ever been in the hospital because of something being wrong with your pancreas? Have you ever been told that you had/have: • Acute pancreatitis? • Chronic pancreatitis?

(*continued*)

(*continued*)

Structure	Question
	If you have been told that you have a pancreas problem, have you had to: • Change your diet? ▪ What foods do you need to avoid? • Avoid all alcohol?
	Have you ever been diagnosed with diabetes? (If so, you can either go into an in-depth assessment of the diagnosis of diabetes now or complete that assessment later. See a later chapter on more information about the assessment of a patient/client with diabetes.)
	Do you take medicine such as enzymes for your pancreas? If so, • What are they? • How often do you have to take them? • Do you take them as prescribed?

SPECIAL SITUATION

The frequency of patients having bariatric surgery for obesity has been consistent. At times, a patient will be referred to telephonic care before/after the surgery to provide ongoing education and support. Should you have a patient who is recovering from bariatric surgery, the following assessment questions might be beneficial.

Before surgery	Would you happen to know your body mass index (BMI)? Or what is your current weight?
	When are you scheduled for the surgery?
	What type of surgery are you going to have?
	What have you been told about the surgery? • Length of hospitalization?
	Do you have any questions about what to expect after the surgery?
	Have you talked with your doctor/health care provider about the questions after the surgery?

(*continued*)

(*continued*)

After surgery	When did you have the procedure?
	How are you feeling right now?
	Have you been back to see the doctor after the surgery?
	How successful has it been so far? Such as: • How much of a weight loss have you experienced?
	Are you having any problems from the surgery?
	How much food would you say you are currently able to eat?
	Are there any foods that you are unable to eat?
	When are you scheduled to see your doctor/health care provider again?

ALGORITHM FOR ASSESSING THE GASTROINTESTINAL SYSTEM

Similar to other body system assessments, this one is quite lengthy too. If you prefer, you can change the approach and just focus on problem areas. Questions to support this are as follows:

Finding	Action
Nausea/vomiting	Assess for length of time nausea has been present.
	Assess for possible causes such as: • Old/spoiled food • New medication
	Assess what has been done for the nausea such as: • Weak tea • Crackers • Dry toast • Ginger ale
	Assess if vomiting is present. If so, assess what it looks like: • Undigested food • Green in color • Black like coffee grounds • Blood

(*continued*)

(continued)

Finding	Action
	Assess for abdominal pain with the nausea and vomiting.
	Suspect gastrointestinal flu or food poisoning if associated with eating and encourage seeking medical attention.
	Suspect gastrointestinal bleeding if emesis is red or black and coffee ground in appearance. (Emesis green in color is bile and not associated with any particular health problem.)
	Suspect small bowel obstruction if nausea is unrelenting and associated with loud audible bowel sounds.
	Encourage to seek immediate medical attention for emesis that is red or black coffee ground in appearance.
Epigastric burning	Assess for pain around the sternum or upper abdomen.
	Assess for when the pain occurs: before eating, during, and after eating?
	Assess what has been done to reduce the burning.
	Assess if eating makes the burning worse or better.
	Suspect gastritis if eating improves the burning.
	Suspect duodenal ulceration if burning/pain occurs several hours after eating.
	Encourage to seek medical attention for evaluation of the epigastric burning.
Diarrhea	Assess for length of time diarrhea has been occurring: number of episodes, number of days.
	Assess for any associated symptoms: gurgling, nausea, and vomiting.
	Assess for color and consistency of stool.
	Assess for presence of blood, mucus, or undigested food in the stool.

(continued)

(continued)

Finding	Action
	Suspect gastrointestinal infection for unexplained onset of diarrhea and encourage to seek medical attention.
Constipation	Assess for last bowel movement.
	Assess for routine bowel movement pattern.
	Assess appearance of stool.
	Assess for any leaking of stool or liquid stool. (Leaking of liquid stool could indicate an impaction.)
	Assess for changes in diet, fluid intake, or activity to contribute to the development of constipation.
	Assess if prescribed opioid analgesics. If so, • The name of the medication • Length of time taking the medication
	Assess what has been done to self-treat the constipation and if it has been effective.
	Assess for routine dietary intake, specifically for foods high in roughage.
	Suspect bowel impaction if leaking of stool or brown-colored fluid is occurring.
	Suspect constipation caused by diet/activity/fluids if a change in oral intake has occurred.
	Suspect opioid-induced constipation if prescribed opioid analgesics.
	Encourage to discuss constipation with doctor/health care provider before ongoing use of over-the-counter laxatives.
Abdominal pain	Assess for location of pain. • Right lower quadrant (suspect appendicitis) • Left lower quadrant (suspect diverticulitis/ diverticulosis) • Mid-abdomen around umbilicus (suspect acute pancreatitis)
	Assess for length of time pain has been occurring.

(continued)

(continued)

Finding	Action
	Assess for what makes the pain worse. What makes it better? (If sitting up or bringing the knees to the abdomen makes the pain better, suspect acute pancreatitis and suggest to seek immediate medical attention.)
	Assess for last bowel movement.
	Assess for associated factors such as: ● After eating ● Ingesting alcohol ● Upon having a bowel movement ● With activity ● Fever ● Nausea/vomiting ● Diarrhea
	Assess for abdomen feeling "bloated" or "swollen."
	Suspect acute abdomen, if right lower quadrant pain and suggest to seek immediate medical attention.
	Suspect a flair of diverticulosis/diverticulitis if associated with eating certain foods and encourage to discuss the health problem with the doctor or health care professional.
Jaundice	Assess where the yellow color is most obvious: sclera of the eyes, palms of the hands, soles of the feet, and skin.
	Assess how long the color has been present.
	Assess if the skin is itchy or any other symptoms.
	Assess for a change in the color of bowel movements.
	Assess if associated with: ● Nausea/vomiting ● Anorexia ● Fatigue ● Fever
	Suspect hepatitis if associated with nausea/vomiting, anorexia, fatigue, and fever and encourage to seek immediate medical attention.

(continued)

(*continued*)

Finding	Action
Rectal bleeding	Assess for when the bleeding started.
	Assess if the bleeding is coating the bowel movement or present on toilet tissue.
	Assess if the bleeding is associated with any abdominal or rectal pain.
	Assess if diagnosed with hemorrhoids.
	Assess how long the bleeding has been occurring.
	Suspect colon pathology if bleeding nonpainful and encourage to seek immediate medical attention.
	Suspect hemorrhoids if bleeding associated with burning/itching/throbbing pain and encourage to seek medical attention.
Right shoulder pain	Assess for approximate location of the pain.
	Assess for length of time the pain has been occurring.
	Assess for when the pain is most noticeable such as after ingesting a large meal with a high-fat content.
	Assess what makes the pain better.
	Assess for changes in bowel pattern or appearance of stool (suspect cholecystitis or cholelithiasis if stool is clay colored).
	Suspect gallbladder disease and encourage to seek medical attention.

See Chapter 15 for additional information about gastrointestinal system disorders

TIPS FOR ASSESSING THE GASTROINTESTINAL SYSTEM

- Remember that this is a body system that many people do not like to discuss. Emphasize that all information will be kept confidential.

- Do not assume that older clients' problems with this system are all age related. Normal age-related changes of the gastrointestinal system include change in smell and taste, slower gastric emptying, and slower propulsion of food through the small bowel and colon.
- Ask if the client has made any dietary changes that could have caused the current issue.
- Find out how much water/fluid is ingested every day. Oftentimes an older client may adjust oral fluid intake to prevent nighttime voiding. This could be a reason for a new onset of constipation.
- Diligently assess if the client reports red or coffee-ground emesis or black stools. This could indicate an active or ongoing bleed somewhere throughout the gastrointestinal tract that needs to be thoroughly investigated.
- Be sure to include asking if the client has any pain that might not seem to be related to the stomach or bowels such as shoulder pain caused by gallbladder disease.
- When asking about weight, find out if the patient has had any changes (gains or losses) that would not be associated with oral intake. If a weight loss is reported, find out if it has been intentional. The patient/client may be following a restricted eating plan with the desired effect of weight loss.

PRACTICE EXERCISES

Read the following client situations and determine:

- Which questions to ask
- What the client might be experiencing
- If the situation is an emergency or should be followed up by a health care professional

1. A member of a wellness program asks if it is normal for abdominal pain to occur after eating nuts and pumpkin seeds.
2. During a routine care call, the patient/client asks what it might mean for there to be drops of blood in the commode after having a bowel movement.

3. A client with a history of bariatric surgery notices an increase in loose runny stools after eating most meals associated with scattered amounts of abdominal pain.

4. During an engagement call, a client in a wellness program asks what over-the-counter laxative would be the best to use since changing to a high-protein, low-carbohydrate eating plan.

5. A client who has been discharged from a substance abuse program asks what it means when the "whites of the eyes" are yellow.

6. After denying abdominal pain a client asks why the right shoulder is so sore.

7. During an assessment, a client makes a comment about the quality of food ingested because the bowel movements are "so skinny" and much lighter in color than usual.

8. A client with a history of small bowel obstruction asks if it is normal to not have a bowel movement for 5 days.

9. While assessing oral intake history, a client states that no alcohol is ingested because it causes severe mid-abdominal pain that lasts for several days.

10. A client asks if it is normal to have diarrhea for several days and then not have a bowel movement for a week but then experiences diarrhea again.

CASE STUDY

Xenia, a telephonic nurse, is preparing to contact a member newly enrolled in a wellness program. She notes that the client has had both an upper and lower gastrointestinal series done the previous year and is prescribed antispasmodic medication.

- On which area of the gastrointestinal system should the assessment focus?
- Why is it essential to ask about the outcome of the gastrointestinal testing?

After introducing the purpose of the program and the frequency of the calls, Xenia finds out that the client has a history of irritable bowel disease.

- What would you like to know about the frequency of bowel movements?
- Why is it important to ask about the characteristics of the stool?

The client reports taking an antispasmodic medication more often than it is prescribed because of so much diarrhea and asks if it would be appropriate to take an over-the-counter medication with it.

- How should this question be answered?
- What direction should you provide to the client?

The client says that when constipation occurs, bowel movements are painful and they are associated with shooting abdominal pain and loud intestinal gurgling.

- What should you suspect is occurring with the client?
- What direction should you provide at this time?

The client agrees to have calls once a week, but is concerned about the employer finding out about the health problem because of a fear of being terminated.

- What should you say to allay the client's fears?
- At which time would it be appropriate to share any personal health information with an employer?

KEY POINTS

- The gastrointestinal system includes many structures, beginning with the mouth, ending with the anus, and including the liver, gallbladder, and pancreas.
- Because a problem can exist anywhere along this tract, the assessment can be quite lengthy.
- Start the assessment with asking if the patient/client is experiencing any particular problem with weight, digestion, or elimination.
- Remember that at no time should an over-the-counter preparation be advised or encouraged. Patients/clients should be referred to their health care provider for treatment.

- If an acute situation is suspected, strongly urge the patient/client to seek immediate medical attention. Symptoms of a gastrointestinal bleed vary greatly. Some patients/clients may experience mild nausea and vomiting, while others may have acute bleeding through emesis or the rectum.
- Do not minimize any older patient's/client's symptoms. Not all gastrointestinal issues are age-related. Changes from what the patient/client considers as being "normal" should be investigated.
- Should any patient/client be edentulous, focus on the ability to ingest food and the type. This could help determine if an associated bowel issue is related to the ability to ingest food instead of another health problem.
- Remember to take your time and ask appropriate questions based on the patient's/client's symptoms. If a problem is not occurring with any particular area, pass on the questions and focus only on those that provide the best information to help improve the patient's/client's health status.

BIBLIOGRAPHY

D'Amico, D., & Barbarito, C. (2012). *Health and physical assessment in nursing* (2nd ed.). Upper Saddle River, NJ: Pearson.

Lemone, P. (2015). *Medical–surgical nursing* (6th ed.). Upper Saddle River, NJ: Pearson.

Pearson Education. (2015). *Nursing: A concept-based approach to learning* (2nd ed., Vol. 2). Upper Saddle River, NJ: Author.

CHAPTER 9

Musculoskeletal System

Upon completion of this chapter, the nurse will:

1. Outline the areas to include when assessing the musculoskeletal system
2. Identify appropriate questions to assess the musculoskeletal system
3. Analyze approaches to gather more information about the musculoskeletal system

THE MUSCULOSKELETAL SYSTEM

The musculoskeletal system includes the bones, joints, cartilage, ligaments, tendons, and muscles found within the body. Bones are identified according to shape, such as:

- Long
- Short
- Flat
- Irregular

The joints are where the bones meet and are categorized as being:

- Cartilaginous
- Fibrous
- Synovial

Cartilage is found between some bones and joints. Ligaments hold bones together.

The muscles within the human body are categorized as being either voluntary or involuntary. Tendons attach muscle to the bones.

ASSESSMENT OVERVIEW

As you might have realized by now, assessment of some of the body systems telephonically has particular challenges. The musculoskeletal system does also. You will not be able to:

- Inspect:
  - Bone structure
  - Posture
  - Spinal structure
  - Gait
  - Range of motion
- Palpate:
  - Muscle tone
  - Muscle strength
  - Joint edema
  - Soft tissue swelling

You will need to use thoughtfully crafted questions to gain as much information as possible when conducting an assessment of the musculoskeletal system over the telephone. As with all of the body systems, the best approach is to ask the patient/client generally, "are you having or have you had any problems with your bones, joints, or muscles?" Depending on the response, you can plan and complete your assessment accordingly.

QUESTIONS TO ASSESS THE MUSCULOSKELETAL SYSTEM

To reduce redundancy, it is recommended that questions about the bones, muscles, and joints be grouped according to body location instead of asking all of the questions about the bones, then repeating the body areas for the muscles and joints.

Body Area	Question
Head	Are you having any problems moving your jaw? • If so, when did this start? • What is the problem? • Does it affect your ability to chew or eat food?

(continued)

(*continued*)

Body Area	Question
	• Is your jaw making a clicking noise? (checking for crepitus) • Have you talked with your doctor or health care provider about your jaw?
Neck	Are you having any problems moving your neck? • If so, when did this start? • What is the problem? • Have you talked with your doctor or health care provider about your neck? • Did you ever have surgery on your neck? ▪ If so, when was it done? ▪ What was the reason for the surgery? • Are you able to bend your head down toward your chest? (flexion) • Are you able to bend your head back and look toward the ceiling? (extension) • Can you move your head to the right? (rotation) • Can you move your head to the left? (rotation) • Can you move your head to try to touch your right shoulder with your right ear? (lateral bending) • Can you move your head to try to touch your left shoulder with your left ear? (lateral bending)
Shoulders	Are you able to freely move your arms from the shoulder? • If not, what is the problem? • When did this start? • Have you talked with your doctor/health care provider about your shoulders? • Did you ever have surgery on your shoulders? ▪ If so, when was it done? ▪ What was the reason for the surgery? • Are you able to lift or carry things on the side that is affected? • Are you able to shrug your shoulders (lift your shoulders toward your ears)? • Can you lift your arms toward the ceiling? (extension) • Can you touch your hands together behind your back? (internal rotation)

(*continued*)

(*continued*)

Body Area	Question
	● Can you place both of your hands behind your neck? (external rotation) ● When standing up can you touch your left thigh with your right hand? (adduction) ● When standing up can you touch your right thigh with your left hand? (adduction) ● Are your shoulders making a clicking or any other type of noise when you move them? (checking for crepitus) ● Have you talked with your doctor or health care provider about your shoulders?
Elbows	Are you able to stretch out your arms? (extension) ● If not, what is the problem? ● When did this start? ● Have you talked with your doctor or health care provider about your elbows? ● Did you ever have surgery on your elbows? 　▪ If so, when was it done? 　▪ What was the reason for the surgery? ● Can you bend your arm at your elbow and touch your hand to your shoulder? (flexion) Are you having any arm weakness? ● If so, when did this start? ● How much are you able to hold and carry with your arms? ● Is one arm weaker than the other?
Wrists and hands	Are you having any problems with your wrists or hands? ● If so, when did this start? ● What is the problem? ● Have you talked with your doctor or health care provider about your wrists and hands? ● Did you ever have surgery on your wrists or hands? 　▪ If so, when was it done? 　▪ What was the reason for the surgery? ● Are you having: 　▪ Weakness 　▪ Numbness 　▪ Tingling ● Can you spread out your fingers? ● Can you make a fist? ● Have your hands or wrists changed in shape?

(*continued*)

(*continued*)

Body Area	Question
	● Can you bend your hand toward the floor from the wrist?
	● Are you able to pick up items with your hands?
	● Can you "feel" your fingers?
	● Do you drop things because of a hand problem?
Hips	Do you have any problems with your hips?
	● If so, what is the problem?
	● When did it start?
	● Does it affect one hip or both?
	● Have you talked with your doctor or health care provider about your hips?
	● Did you ever have surgery on your hips?
	▪ If so, when was it done?
	▪ What was the reason for the surgery?
	● Does the skin over your hips feel warm?
	● Do your hips make a grating or clicking sound when you walk? (crepitus)
	● Do you have pain in your hips when you:
	▪ Walk
	▪ Sit
	▪ Cross the legs (adduction)
	● Can you stretch out your leg at the hip? (extension)
	● Can you raise your knees toward your chest? (flexion)
	● Can you move your right leg out to the side? (abduction)
	● Can you move your left leg out to the side? (abduction)
Knees	Do you have any problems with your knees?
	● If so, what is the problem?
	● Have you talked with your doctor or health care provider about your knees?
	● Did you ever have surgery on your knees?
	▪ If so, when was it done?
	▪ What was the reason for the surgery?
	● When did it start?
	● Does it affect one knee or both?
	● Does the skin over the knees feel warm?
	● Does the tissue around the knee feel swollen?
	● Can you bend your right knee? (flexion)
	● Can you bend your left knee? (flexion)

(*continued*)

(*continued*)

Body Area	Question

Ankles and feet	Do you have any problems with your ankles?
	• If so, what is the problem?
	• Are your ankles swollen?
	• Is the skin around your ankles red?
	• Do your ankles hurt when you walk?
	• Have you talked with your doctor or health care provider about your ankles?
	• Did you ever have surgery on your ankles?
	  ▪ If so, when was it done?
	  ▪ What was the reason for the surgery?
	• Are you able to move your feet toward the floor (push down on the gas pedal)? (extension)
	• Are you able to point your toes toward the ceiling? (flexion)
	Do you have any problems with your feet or toes?
	• If so, what is the problem?
	• Have you talked with your doctor or health care provider about your feet or toes?
	• Did you ever have surgery on your feet or toes?
	  ▪ If so, when was it done?
	  ▪ What was the reason for the surgery?
	• Are any of your toes swollen?
	• Are any of your toes not straight?
	• Do any of your toes overlap?
	• Do you have any sores on your feet or toes?
	• Are you able to curl your toes toward the floor? (flexion)
	• Are you able to spread your toes out? (extension)

Spine	Do you have any problems with your back?
	• If so, what is the problem?
	• When did it start?
	• Have you talked with your doctor or health care provider about your back?
	• Did you ever have surgery on your back?
	  ▪ If so, when was it done?
	  ▪ What was the reason for the surgery?
	• Are you able to walk?
	• Do you use anything to keep yourself stable when you walk like a:
	  ▪ Cane
	  ▪ Walker
	  ▪ Crutches

(*continued*)

(continued)

Body Area	Question
	• Has anyone ever told you that you have one leg longer/shorter than the other?
	• Are you able to bend over and touch the floor with your hands? (flexion)
	• Do you have any pain or stiffness when you straighten your spine after bending over? (extension)
	Do you have any problems keeping your balance?
	• If so, what does it feel like?
	• Have you fallen?
	Have you had a change in your body height?
	• If so, how tall were you?
	• What is your height now?
	• Did your doctor or health care provider tell you why your height has changed?
	Have you ever been told that you have a spinal deformity such as:
	• Lordosis
	• Kyphosis
	• Scoliosis

SPECIAL SITUATIONS

At times, a client may be enrolled in a disease management program for arthritis or other musculoskeletal system disorder and be home recovering from surgery. Suggestions to help with the assessment of these clients are as follows:

Situation	Question
Hip replacement or other hip surgery	When did you have the surgery?
	What did you have done?
	Are you able to walk or bear any weight on the leg that was operated on?
	What are you using to make sure that you walk safely?
	What does the wound/incision look like?

(continued)

(continued)

Situation	Question
	Are you experiencing any problems such as: • Increased pain • Drainage from the surgical wound • Increased swelling around the surgical wound • Fever
	When are you going to see your surgeon again?
	Are you getting physical therapy at home? • If so, how many times a week?
	Have you been told to avoid doing anything in particular?
	For what reasons did your doctor/health care provider tell you to contact the office?
Knee replacement or other knee surgery	When did you have the surgery?
	What did you have done?
	Are you able to walk or bear any weight on the leg that was operated on?
	What are you using to make sure that you walk safely?
	What does the wound/incision look like?
	Are you experiencing any problems such as: • Increased pain • Drainage from the surgical wound • Increased swelling around the surgical wound • Fever
	When are you going to see your surgeon again?
	Are you getting physical therapy at home? • If so, how many times a week? • Are you doing your knee-bending exercises as instructed?
	Have you been told to avoid doing anything in particular?

(continued)

(continued)

Situation	Question
	For what reasons did your doctor or health care provider tell you to contact the office?
Spinal/back surgery	When did you have the surgery?
	What did you have done?
	Are you able to walk without any pain or discomfort?
	Are you supposed to: ● Wear a back brace ● Walk with a cane/walker
	Are you permitted to take a shower?
	Are you experiencing any problems such as: ● Increased pain ● Drainage from the surgical wound ● Increased swelling around the surgical wound ● Fever
	When are you going to see your surgeon again?
	Are you being visited by a home care nurse?
	Have you been told to avoid doing anything in particular?
	For what reasons did your doctor or health care provider tell you to contact the office?

ALGORITHM FOR ASSESSING THE MUSCULOSKELETAL SYSTEM

At times, you might be placing a call to a patient who is experiencing a new onset of symptoms. Suggestions for these situations are as follows:

Finding	Action
Pain	Assess for the location of the pain.
	Assess the level of pain using the standard 0–10 pain rating scale.

(continued)

(continued)

Finding	Action
	Assess for what might have caused the pain: • Recent fall
	Assess what has been done to treat the pain
	Assess for any other associated symptoms such as: • Inability to walk without severe pain (fracture or dislocation) • Sudden shortening of one leg (dislocated or fractured hip)
	Suspect fracture or dislocation and encourage to seek immediate medical attention.
Swollen joint	Assess the location of the joint
	Assess for the length of time the joint has been swollen
	Assess what has been done to try to relieve the swelling: • Elevate on a pillow • Wrap with an elastic bandage • Apply ice
	Assess the color of the skin over the joint: • Red • Bruised
	Assess for any other symptoms: • Fever • Nausea • Vomiting
	Assess if there has been any change in ability to perform activities of daily living because of the swollen joint
	Suspect acute joint inflammation and encourage to seek medical attention
Crepitus	Assess for the joint causing the crepitus
	Assess for the length of time the crepitus has been occurring
	Assess if the crepitus is associated with any pain
	Suspect no acute disease process
	Encourage to discuss the "noises" during the patient's next visit to the doctor or health care provider

(continued)

(*continued*)

Finding	Action
Numbness/ tingling	Assess for the location of the numbness/tingling
	Assess for the length of time the numbness/tingling has been occurring
	Assess what has been done to try to alleviate the numbness/tingling: • Elevating legs • Removing compression stockings or gloves • Rubbing the hands/feet
	Assess for any other associated symptoms such as: • New onset of limb weakness (stroke) • Confusion (stroke) • Blurred vision (stroke) • Pain (acute venous or arterial occlusion) • Skin over the area feels cold to the touch (acute venous or arterial occlusion)
	Suspect an acute situation and encourage the patient to seek immediate medical attention
Muscle cramping/ muscle spasms	Assess for the location of the muscle cramping/spasm
	Assess for the length of time the muscle has been cramping/spasming
	Assess for any activities that cause the cramping/ spasming to occur or change in intensity
	Assess for any other symptoms associated with the cramping/spasming such as: • Nausea (electrolyte imbalance) • Vomiting (electrolyte imbalance) • Diarrhea (electrolyte imbalance)
	Assess what has been done to relieve the cramping/ spasms such as: • Massage • Elevation • Exercise/stretching
	Encourage to discuss cramping/spasms with doctor/ health care provider soon

See Chapter 16 for additional information about musculoskeletal system disorders.

TIPS FOR ASSESSING THE MUSCULOSKELETAL SYSTEM

- Unless the client mentions body "aches and pains," it is unlikely that you will need to complete a full musculoskeletal status assessment.
- Some older clients assume that body "aches and pains" are a normal part of aging and may not want to talk about it.
- Other clients may prefer to spend all of the time on the telephone talking about their "aches and pains." Should this occur, work through the assessment, focusing on the areas in which the patient/client is experiencing difficulty.
- Be sure to find out what actions or activities make the body "aches and pains" better or worse. The pain and stiffness of arthritis can be more severe in the morning and improves with activity.
- If a client experiences numbness and tingling of the hands, be sure to find out what activities are routinely performed. This could indicate carpal tunnel syndrome.
- If any client reports a recent fall, be sure to follow up with questioning about the outcome of a health care provider appointment. Everyone who falls does not seek immediate medical attention, but depending on other health problems, the fall could have caused a break or other tissue injury. If the injury is not treated now, it could cause the patient/client problems in the future.

PRACTICE EXERCISES

Read the following client situations and determine:

- Which questions to ask
- What the client might be experiencing
- If the situation is an emergency or should be followed up by a health care professional

1. A middle-aged female client asks what it means if there is pain near the ear when the mouth is opened to brush the teeth.
2. An older client states that over the last several months, the left side of the neck has been tender to the touch and has not been able to turn the head toward the left shoulder.

3. A member of a wellness program is unable to touch the hands behind the back and experiences sharp pains across the chest when this action is attempted.
4. A client in a disease management program asks what can be done for hand numbness and tingling that started shortly after being instructed to use two canes to walk.
5. An older patient with diabetes fell at home and has noticed tightness in the right leg. The leg seems to be "not as long" as the other one now.
6. A client who works in a factory asks what could be causing cramps in both calves that occur when trying to sleep.
7. A client calls into the office, upset because the right knee made a "cracking" noise and wonders if the bone has broken.
8. A member of a wellness program mentions that the right elbow has been swollen and painful after playing tennis the previous Saturday afternoon.
9. A client with scoliosis notices an increase in lower lumbar back pain after walking while at work for several hours.
10. A client recovering from knee replacement surgery reports tripping over the dog, falling on the operative knee, and unable to bend the leg at the knee.

CASE STUDY

The nurses who work for a health insurance plan are reviewing recent claims submitted by enrollees for services related to the musculoskeletal system.

- What questions would be appropriate to ask when assessing enrollees who had the following claims paid?
  - Wrist and hand x-rays
  - MRI of the spine
  - CT scan of the neck
  - X-rays of the right hip
  - Physical therapy for progressive ambulation
  - Durable medical equipment for elevated commode seat and crutches

The health insurance nurses decide to refer several enrollees to a wellness program for telephonic care.

- What makes these clients at risk for hospitalization for a musculoskeletal-related health problem?
  - 89-year-old female who has lost 4 inches in height over the last decade
  - 50-year-old male who plays golf twice a week
  - 34-year-old female who works as a computer analyst
  - 75-year-old male receiving dialysis for chronic renal failure
  - 82-year-old female with sleep apnea who wears oxygen continuously

The health insurance nurse is making a list of enrollees to telephone to explain their enrollment in the wellness program.

- Why should these clients be referred immediately to a health care provider?
  - 65-year-old enrollee who is experiencing weakness on the left side of the body
  - 28-year-old enrollee who fell during a hiking trip
  - 46-year-old enrollee who works as a pharmaceutical representative and is experiencing a new onset of left shoulder weakness
  - 62-year-old newly retired enrollee experiencing bilateral knee pain after gardening for several hours
  - 70-year-old retired house painter experiencing swelling, pain, and redness of the left ankle

KEY POINTS

- Begin the musculoskeletal system assessment with a general question regarding the patient's/client's physical status.
- Remember that careful questioning will take the place of inspection and palpation of this system.
- Focus the assessment on problem areas first.
- Take your time when providing telephonic care to a patient/client recovering from musculoskeletal surgery. The patient/client could be at risk for postsurgical complications.
- Ask as many questions as needed to obtain as clear a picture as possible about the patient's/client's musculoskeletal status.
- Do not assume that all older patients/clients will experience "aches and pains."

BIBLIOGRAPHY

D'Amico, D., & Barbarito, C. (2012). *Health and physical assessment in nursing* (2nd ed.). Upper Saddle River, NJ: Pearson.

Lemone, P. (2015). *Medical–surgical nursing* (6th ed.). Upper Saddle River, NJ: Pearson.

Pearson Education. (2015). *Nursing: A concept-based approach to learning* (2nd ed., Vol. 2). Upper Saddle River, NJ: Author.

U.S. National Library of Medicine & Medline Plus. (2014). Tendon versus ligament. Retrieved from https://www.nlm.nih.gov/medlineplus/ency/imagepages/19089.htm

CHAPTER 10

Neurologic and Sensory Systems

Upon completion of this chapter, the nurse will:

1. Outline the areas to include when assessing the neurologic and sensory systems
2. Identify appropriate questions to assess the neurologic and sensory systems
3. Analyze approaches to gather more information about the neurologic and sensory systems

THE NEUROLOGIC SYSTEM

For many nurses the neurologic system can be overwhelming because this system interacts and controls all other body systems. As a review, the neurologic system is divided into:

- Central nervous system:
  - Brain
  - Spinal cord
- Peripheral nervous system:
  - Cranial nerves
  - Spinal nerves

Central Nervous System

The Brain

The brain contains the frontal, temporal, parietal, and occipital lobes. Each lobe is responsible for specific body functions.

Lobe	Functions
Frontal	● Voluntary movement ● Speech ● Thinking ● Emotions
Temporal	● Interpretation of hearing ● Sense of smell
Parietal	● Conscious awareness ● Pain ● Temperature
Occipital	● Vision

Additional structures within "the brain" include the following:

Structure	Function
Cerebellum	● Body movement ● Positioning
Diencephalon ● Thalamus ● Hypothalamus	● Autonomic control center to control: ▪ Blood pressure ▪ Heart rate ▪ Respiratory rate ▪ Temperature
Brain stem ● Midbrain ● Pons ● Medulla oblongata	● Site for 10 cranial nerves ● Controls vasoconstriction ● Regulates: ▪ Respiratory depth and rhythm ▪ Coughing ▪ Sneezing ▪ Swallowing

The Spinal Cord

The spinal cord is an extension of the medulla oblongata and ends around the first or second lumbar vertebra. This structure is the relay station for sensory and motor input, and the function is divided into cervical, thoracic, and lumbar sections.

Peripheral Nervous System

Cranial Nerves

Learning the cranial nerves for nursing school was not always an easy feat. There is no need to memorize them now. There are 12 cranial nerves, each with a specific function.

Nerve	Function
I Olfactory	• Smell
II Optic	• Vision
III Oculomotor	• Pupil response • Eye muscle movement
IV Trochlear	• Eye muscle movement
V Trigeminal	• Three branches: ▪ Ophthalmic: eye sensation ▪ Maxillary: lower eyelid, nose, upper teeth, and upper lip ▪ Mandibular: lower teeth, tongue, chin, and lower lip
VI Abducens	• Eye movement
VII Facial	• Taste • Facial movement • Tears • Saliva
VIII Vestibulocochlear	• Two branches: ▪ Vestibular: balance ▪ Cochlear: hearing
IX Glossopharyngeal	• Gag reflex • Swallowing • Taste
X Vagus	• Throat • Swallowing • Receptor responses
XI Accessory	• Trapezius and sternocleidomastoid muscle movement • Inner throat movement
XII Hypoglossal	• Tongue movement to swallow • Chewing • Speech

Spinal Nerves

There are 31 pairs of spinal nerves that correspond to the vertebral level.

Vertebral Level	Nerves
Cervical	Nerves C1–C8
Thoracic	Nerves T1–T12
Lumbar	Nerves L1–L5
Sacral	Nerves S1–S5
Coccygeal	1 nerve

THE SENSORY SYSTEM

The sensory system contains the eyes and ears. Structures of the eye can be divided into three layers:

- Cornea
- Choroid
  - Iris
  - Pupil
- Retina
  - Optic disc
  - Macula

There are three parts to the ears, which include:

- External ear
  - Ear canal
- Middle ear
  - Tympanic membrane
  - Eustachian tubes
- Inner ear
  - Cochlea

ASSESSMENT OVERVIEW

As you can see, the neurologic and sensory systems contain a large number of structures and perform many body functions. You will be challenged to complete these assessments and will be limited in your ability to:

- Observe body movement and positioning
- Assess cranial and spinal nerve functioning
- Determine eye function and pupillary response

The one status that you will be able to assess thoroughly is that of hearing because you will be asking carefully structured, succinct questions in order to determine the functioning of these body systems. As with the previous body systems, the best approach might be to introduce this assessment by saying, "Let's spend some time now talking about the nerves, vision, and hearing. Before we get started, are you having or have you had any problems with your nerves, eyes, or ears?" Plan your assessment according to the response.

QUESTIONS TO ASSESS THE NEUROLOGIC SYSTEM

Body Area	Question
Brain	Have you ever had an injury to your head? If so, • When did this occur? • How was it treated? • Have you had many changes because of the injury?
Frontal lobe	Do you have any problems walking or moving your arms and legs?
	(Observe the patient's speech pattern. You will not be going into an in-depth assessment of thinking/reasoning/judgment but ask about activities of daily living and instrumental activities of daily living.) Are you able to complete your own care needs such as: • Bathing? • Dressing? • Toileting? • Eating? Are you able to perform routine activities such as: • Cooking? • Grocery shopping? • Balancing a checkbook?

(*continued*)

(*continued*)

Body Area	Question
Temporal lobe	Have you had or are you experiencing any changes in your ability to smell things? If so, what are the changes? ● Do you have smoke alarms in your (home, apartment, room)?
	(This lobe is responsible for the interpretation of hearing. If the patient/client is responding appropriately to your questions, it is unlikely that there are any issues with hearing interpretation.) If the patient/client is not responding appropriately to questions: ● Are you able to hear me? . ● Can you understand what I am saying? (Be advised that these are not appropriate questions for a patient with English as a second language or someone who recently relocated to the United States and has not mastered the English language. These questions are to assess if the spoken word is being appropriately transmitted to the temporal lobe for sensory interpretation and not to measure ability to comprehend a different language.)
Parietal lobe	Is the temperature of the room where you sitting right now comfortable to you? ● Is it too hot, too cold? ● Are you able to adjust your clothing or environment if it is too hot or too cold?
	Are you having any pain right now? If so, ● Where is the pain? ● Describe what it feels like. ● How long does it last? ● What makes it better? ● What makes it worse?
Occipital lobe	Although we will spend more time on vision shortly, can you tell me if you have or have had any problems with your vision? ● Tell me some of the items around you right now.
Additional brain structures	Do you have any problems swallowing?

(*continued*)

(*continued*)

Body Area	Question
	Do you ever feel like you aren't stable on your feet when standing still or walking?
	Do you have or have you had any issues with a cough or sneezing?
Cranial nerves	(If no issue with sense of smell, no need to repeat asking questions about CN I)
	(If no issue with vision, no need to repeat asking questions about CN II, III, IV, and VI)
	Do you have or have you had any problems with pain on the skin around your eyes, cheeks, or jaw? If so, ● Is the pain constant? ● Is it aggravated by something else, such as eating, drinking, talking, smoking, or cold air? ● What makes the pain better? ● Have you been treated for this face pain? If so, ● What is/was the treatment/medication? ● How often do you use the treatment/medication?
	When you smile do both sides of your mouth move? If not, which side does not move? ● How long has this been going on?
	Do you have any problems swallowing food or liquids? If so, ● What is the problem? How long has this been going on?
	Have you had or are you having any problems with the taste of food? If so, ● What foods taste different? ● What is the taste that you are experiencing? ● How long has this been going on?
	Have you had or are you having any problems chewing food? If so, ● What is the problem? ● How long has this been going on?

(*continued*)

(*continued*)

Body Area	Question
	Have you had or are you having any problems with your tongue? If so, • Describe the problem. • How long has this been going on?
Spinal nerves	Are you having or have you had any pain that was caused by nerve irritation? Such as: • Neck pain • Arm pain • Pain down the back of your leg • Lower back pain • Foot pain If so, • When does the pain occur? • What makes it better? • What makes it worse? • What have you been told about the pain?
	Have you had an injury to your neck or back at any time? If so, • What was the injury? • When did it happen? • How was it treated? • How does it feel right now? • Is there anything that you have to do now to prevent it from happening again?
	Have you had or currently have numbness or tingling of any body part. If so, • Where is the numbness/tingling occurring? • How long does it last? • What makes it better? • What makes it worse? • What have you been told about the numbness/tingling?
	Have you ever had any operations on your neck or back? If so, • What was done? • When was it done? • Why was it done?

(*continued*)

(*continued*)

Body Area	Question
	Have you had or currently have weakness of any arms or legs? If so, ● Which arm/leg? ● On the right side of the body? ● On the left side of the body? ● How long has this been going on? ● What has your doctor/health care provider told you about the weakness? Has the weakness changed your ability to: ● Walk? ● Eat? ● Perform other activities?
Eyes	Do you have any problems seeing/with your vision? If so, what is the problem? ● Blurred vision ● Blind spots ● Floaters
	Do you wear eyeglasses? For what reason? ● All of the time ● To read ● For distance ● When driving
	Have you ever been told that you have an eye problem such as: ● Glaucoma? ● Cataracts (cloudy vision)? ● Macular degeneration (loss of central vison)?
	Have you ever had eye surgery? If so, what was it for? ● Detached retina ● Laser surgery (to correct vision) ● Laser surgery (to stop bleeding from diabetic retinopathy)
	Are you prescribed any medications for your eyes? If so, ● What is the name of the medicine? ● How many drops each time? ● How often are they used? ● What are they for?

(*continued*)

(*continued*)

Body Area	Question
	Do you have any problems with: ● Eye tearing? ● Dry eyes?
	How often do you see your eye doctor? ● When is your next appointment?
Ears	Are you having any problems with your ears right now? If so, ● What is the problem? ● Is the problem "buzzing" or "ringing" in the ears? ● How long has it been going on? ● What have you been doing about it?
	How do you remove wax from your ears?
	Are you having any problems with your hearing? If so, ● How long has this been going on? ● Do you use a hearing aid? ● What kind of hearing aid do you have?
	Have you ever had surgery on your ears? If so, ● When was it done? ● What was it for? ● Did the surgery fix the problem?

ALGORITHM FOR ASSESSING THE NEUROLOGIC AND SENSORY SYSTEMS

If you are calling a patient/client who is experiencing a new set of symptoms, the following questions might be helpful.

Finding	Action
Headache	Assess for the location of the headache: ● At the base of the neck (hypertension) ● Top of the head ● Temporal area ● Forehead (sinus) ● Behind the eyes (cluster, sinus)

(*continued*)

(continued)

Finding	Action
	Assess for when the headache started: ● Woke up with it in the morning (hypertension) ● Gradually during the day (migraine, tension) ● After sitting and working at a computer (tension)
	Assess for any other symptoms: ● Eye pain with light (photophobia) ● Eye tearing (cluster headache) ● Nausea/vomiting (increasing intracranial pressure, Meniere's disease)
	Suspect: ● Headache associated with hypertension (assess further if patient/client has a history of this disorder) ● Tension headache if occurs after sitting/working in a hunched position ● Sinus headache if associated with forehead pain, nasal stuffiness ● Migraine headache if associated with photophobia ● Cluster headache if associated with eye tearing ● Increasing intracranial pressure if associated with nausea/vomiting: ■ Assess for changes in level of responsiveness ● Meniere's disease if associated with nausea/vomiting: ■ Assess for hearing and dizziness
	Encourage to seek medical attention for any new onset of symptoms
Pain	Assess for location of pain: ● Eye ● Leg ● Ear ● Back
	Assess for when the pain started: ● After reading ● Sitting ● Walking ● Lifting an object or twisting

(continued)

(*continued*)

Finding	Action
	Assess for length of time pain has been occurring
	Assess for what has been done to help the pain
	Assess for any associated symptoms: • Acute loss of vision (acute glaucoma, detached retina) • Loss of hearing (ruptured eardrum) • Limb numbness/tingling/weakness (nerve compression)
	Suspect: • Acute onset glaucoma, detached retina with loss of vision • Acute onset ruptured tympanic membrane with loss of hearing • Nerve compression with limb numbness/tingling/weakness
	Encourage to seek medical attention for any new onset of symptoms
Change in vision	Assess for the change: • Complete loss of vision in one/both eyes • Loss of peripheral vision • Loss of central vision • Blurred vision • Spots in vision • Cloudy vision • "Yellow haze" or "halo" vision
	Assess for length of time vision change has occurred: • Sudden • Gradual • Upon waking up in the morning • Over the course of the day
	Assess for any associated symptoms: • Eye pain • Tearing • Eye drainage/mucus • "Red" eyes

(*continued*)

(continued)

Finding	Action
	Suspect: • Acute onset glaucoma with eye pain • Macular degeneration with loss of central vision • Glaucoma with loss of peripheral vision • Cataracts with cloudy vision • Floaters with "spots" in vision • Medication adverse effect (digitalis/digoxin) with yellow or halo vision • Infection with red eyes and drainage • Metabolic disorder (diabetes) with blurred vision (Conduct additional assessments if indicated)
	Encourage to seek medical attention for any new onset of symptoms
Ears Ringing (Tinnitus)/Acute onset of deafness	Assess when the ear ringing/deafness started (Assess medications if noticed after starting/taking a specific medication such as ototoxic antibiotics or over-the-counter aspirin)
	Assess activities being done when the ear ringing/deafness started: • Listening to loud music • Loud bang/gunshot/bomb • Swimming/water in the ears • Cleaning the ears with an ear swab or other object
	Assess for any other symptoms: • Nausea/vomiting • Pain in or around the ear • Drainage/bleeding from the ear
	Suspect: • Acute irritation if occurring after loud music, loud noise • Acute ear infection if associated with water in the ears/swimming • Tympanic membrane rupture if associated with cleaning the ears • Medication adverse effect if associated with medications
	Encourage to seek medical attention for any new onset of symptoms

(continued)

(*continued*)

Finding	Action
Onset of paralysis	Access if paralysis is on one side (both arm and leg) or just one limb
	Assess when the paralysis started
	Suspect acute stroke and refer for immediate medical attention

See **Chapter 17** *for additional information about neurologic and sensory system disorders.*

TIPS FOR ASSESSING THE NEUROLOGIC AND SENSORY SYSTEMS

- Begin the assessment with asking if the client has experienced any new changes or symptoms.
- Use terms such as "feeling" or "numbness" to describe a problem with the cranial and/or peripheral nerves. Clients may become confused if the term "nerves" is used and think the assessment will focus on "nervousness" or "anxiety."
- An acute onset of any new symptom should be investigated immediately.
- Any onset of slurred speech or confusion could indicate a stroke. Obtain medical assistance for the client.
- Emphasize that any acute change in vision or hearing needs immediate attention. Acute loss of vision in one eye could indicate a detached retina, requiring immediate surgery.
- Take the time and further assess any symptoms that might be attributed to a problem in another body system.

PRACTICE EXERCISES

Read the following client situations and determine:

- Which questions to ask.
- What the client might be experiencing.
- If the situation is an emergency or should be followed up by a health care professional.

1. A young adult in a wellness program asks if it is "normal" to feel dizzy and nauseated after falling off of a skateboard and hitting the head.
2. A middle-aged adult mentions progressive cloudiness of vision in the right eye.
3. An older client says that hearing has been getting progressively worse ever since starting on medicine to treat a "chest cold."
4. During a routine call, a member asks "what it means" if the right arm and leg are both numb and tingling at the same time.
5. After explaining the purpose of care calls a client says that her left lower leg and foot have been numb "for years."
6. A middle-aged client explains that pain "behind the eyes" has been going on "for days" but now the one eye is tearing.
7. An older client says that food has lost its flavor and needs to add "tons" of salt before eating.
8. A middle-aged client asks why the vision would be blurry "just in the middle."
9. An older client says that his hearing must be getting worse because the hearing aids don't seem to be working any more.
10. A middle-aged client asks what would cause the face "to hurt."

CASE STUDY

Allie, a telephonic nurse, is scheduled to make a care call to a new member enrolled in the disease management program for heart disease. Prior to making the call, Allie reviews the most recent claims paid for diagnostic tests and medications.

- Why is it important to consider conducting a neurologic system assessment with this member?
- On which areas should you focus the assessment?

The member agrees to be in the program and apologizes for the slurred speech saying it has been becoming worse over the last few hours.

- What might be occurring with this member?
- What should you do?

After ensuring the member is taken for medical attention, Allie schedules a follow-up call for 1 week. When making the call a week later, Allie is told that the member is "unavailable" and to call back in a month.

- What should you suspect has happened with this client?
- What might have been done before ending the last call?

Allie searches through claims information and learns that the member is currently in a rehabilitation facility. The expected length of stay is 28 days.

- When calling back in a month, what safety issues should you focus on?
- What potential issues with nutrition and communication should be explored?

KEY POINTS

- The neurologic and sensory systems are intertwined with other major body systems.
- Telephonic assessment of the neurologic system depends on whether the patient/client is experiencing any symptoms.
- Any acute symptom needs to be further investigated. Use your best judgment. If the patient/client is experiencing acute blindness/hearing loss/paralysis or other manifestations of a stroke, do not delay obtaining medical attention.
- Not all symptoms are life-threatening. If the patient/client does not sound to be in acute distress, take few extra minutes and conduct further assessment.

BIBLIOGRAPHY

D'Amico, D., & Barbarito, C. (2012). *Health and physical assessment in nursing* (2nd ed.). Upper Saddle River, NJ: Pearson.

Lemone, P. (2015). *Medical-surgical nursing* (6th ed.). Upper Saddle River, NJ: Pearson.

Pearson Education. (2015). *Nursing: A concept-based approach to learning* (2nd ed., Vol. 1). Upper Saddle River, NJ: Author.

CHAPTER 11

Genitourinary System

LEARNING OUTCOMES

Upon completion of this chapter, the nurse will:

1. Outline the areas to include when assessing the genitourinary system
2. Identify appropriate questions to assess the genitourinary system
3. Analyze approaches to gather more information about the genitourinary system

THE GENITOURINARY SYSTEM

The genitourinary system contains the systems needed to produce urine, the process of urination, and reproductive organs. For both males and females, the urinary system includes:

- Kidneys
- Ureters
- Bladder
- Urethra

For the female reproductive system, the organs include:

- Breasts
- Ovaries
- Fallopian tubes
- Uterus
- Cervix
- Vagina

And for the male reproductive system, the organs include:

- Prostate
- Testes
- Penis

ASSESMENT OVERVIEW

Other than renal failure, the number of clients enrolled in a disease management or wellness program having a primary problem involving the genitourinary system will be minimal. It is more likely for clients to have issues with this body system in addition to another health problem. Similar to the other body systems, the techniques to assess this system are limited. You will not be able to:

- Observe urine color
- Observe skin color
- Palpate skin turgor
- Palpate for bladder distention
- Palpate the breasts
- Percuss the kidneys
- Auscultate for renal blood flow

This body system is inherently private. Many clients will not want to discuss issues with urine output or problems with reproductive organs. Your assessment questions, at times, may seem vague; however, using this approach reduces involuntary client resistance to providing assessment information.

A general question to begin the assessment of this body system might be "do you have any problems passing urine/water?" This can be followed by "are you able to make it to the bathroom in time to empty your bladder?" For an older female client, asking about children would be an appropriate opening to assess the reproductive system. For an older male client, a general question such as "have you ever been told you have a problem with your prostate or other private body parts" is less intrusive. Then, plan your assessment according to the responses.

QUESTIONS TO ASSESS THE GENITOURINARY SYSTEM

Body Area	Question
Kidneys/Ureters	Have you ever had a problem with your kidneys? If so, what was the problem? ● Kidney stones ● Renal failure
	How was/is the problem being treated? ● Lithotripsy ● Other treatment ● Dialysis
	Have you had to change your diet or fluid intake because of: ● Kidney stones? ● Dialysis?
	What medicines are you taking specifically for the: ● Kidney stones? ● Dialysis?
	Are you having/or had changes in your skin? If so, ● Is your skin drier/moist? ● Has it changed in color (for example, does it look more yellow)? ● Does it feels itchy?
Bladder/Urethra	How often do you go to the bathroom to urinate?
	What does your urine look like? Is it: ● Clear? ● Yellow? ● Cloudy? ● Dark (like tea)? ● Pink (blood-tinged)?
	Are you able to make it to the bathroom to urinate?
	Do you ever wake up in the middle of the night to urinate? If so, ● How many times each night?
	Do you ever have a problem starting to urinate?

(continued)

(continued)

Body Area	Question
	Do you ever feel like you still have urine in your bladder after going to the bathroom?
	Do you ever experience: • Burning? • Pain? When urinating? If so, • How often does this occur? • What have you done about it?
Female reproductive: Breasts	When was your last mammogram? (This will depend on the age of the client.)
	Do you routinely examine your breasts? If so, • How often?
	Have you ever had a problem with your breasts? If so, what was the problem? • Cysts • Cancer
	How was your breast problem treated? • Draining of the cysts • Biopsy • Surgery/chemotherapy/radiation (cancer)
Ovaries/Fallopian tubes/Uterus	Are you (still) having regular menstrual periods? If so, • When was your last menstrual period? • If not, when did you stop having menstrual periods?
	Are you experiencing any changes or issues with your menstrual period? or Are you experiencing any changes or issues since not having menstrual periods?
	Have you ever had surgery to your female organs? If so, • When was it done? • What type of surgery was it? • What was it for? Are you having any problems since having the surgery?

(continued)

(*continued*)

Body Area	Question
Cervix/Vagina	When was your last gynecologic (gyne) examination?
	Did you have a Pap smear done? ● Were there any problems with the Pap smear? If so, ▪ What was the problem? ▪ What was the treatment?
	(Depending on the age of the client, this next question might be appropriate.) Have you received the vaccination to prevent the development of cervical cancer? If so, ● When did you receive the vaccination?
	Have you had/do you have any open sores or lumps on the skin around your vagina? If so, ● When does this occur? ● How often does it occur? ● What has been done about the lumps/sores?
Male reproductive: Prostate	Have you ever had a prostate exam? If so, ● When was it done last? ● Were there any problems found?
	Have you ever had a problem with your prostate (gland)? If so, what was the problem? ● Enlarged prostate ● Infection (prostatitis)
	Have you ever had surgery on your prostate gland? If so, do you remember the name of the surgery? ● When was it done?
Testes	Have you had an examination of your testicles? If so, ● When was it done? ● Were there any problems?
	Do you perform a self-examination of your testicles? If so, ● How often?

(*continued*)

(*continued*)

Body Area	Question
	Have you ever had surgery on your testicles? If so, ● What was it for? ● When was it done?
Penis	Have you had any problems with your penis such as: ● Drainage? 　▪ If so, describe the type of drainage 　▪ How often does it occur? ● Open sores? 　▪ If so, where are they located? 　▪ What is done to help them heal? What have you been told about the drainage/open sores? ● What is the cause?
	Do you have any problems with intimacy (this is one way of asking if the male client is able to have an erection)? If so, ● How long has this been going on? ● What has been done about it? ● Do you take medication for it?

ALGORITHM FOR ASSESSING THE GENITOURINARY SYSTEM

If you are calling a patient/client who is experiencing a new set of symptoms, the following questions might be helpful:

Finding	Action
Blood in the urine	Assess for urine color such as: ● Frank red blood ● Pink tinged
	Assess for presence of pain with bleeding
	Assess for location of pain with bleeding such as: ● Side of the back (flank pain) ● Groin ● Urethra

(*continued*)

(continued)

Finding	Action
	Assess for any other symptoms such as: ● Nausea/vomiting ● Fever
	For hematuria associated with pain, suspect a urinary tract infection or kidney stone.
	For painless hematuria, suspect undiagnosed neoplasm.
	Encourage to seek medical attention for any new onset of symptoms.
Dark urine	Assess for color such as: ● Tea colored ● Cola colored
	Assess for associated symptoms such as: ● Flank pain ● Foam in the urine
	Assess for changes in fluid intake
	Suspect dehydration, kidney stone, or renal failure
	Encourage to seek medical attention for any new onset of symptoms
Flank pain	Assess for length of time pain has been occurring
	Assess for associated symptoms such as: ● Change in urine output ● Characteristics of urine (mucous threads, pus, blood) ● Groin pain
	Suspect kidney stone
	Encourage to seek medical attention for any new onset of symptoms
Burning with urination	Assess for length of time burning has been occurring

(continued)

(continued)

Finding	Action
	Assess for urine characteristics to include: • Dark urine • Blood in urine • Pus/mucus in urine
	Assess for other symptoms such as: • Flank pain • Fever
	Suspect a urinary tract infection
	Encourage to seek medical attention for any new onset of symptoms
No urine output	Assess for length of time since the last voiding occurred
	Assess for associated symptoms such as: • Edema of the feet/ankles/hands/around the eyes • Itchy skin • Change in skin color • Nausea/vomiting • Flank or groin pain
	Suspect kidney stone or acute onset of renal failure
	Encourage to seek medical attention for any new onset of symptoms
Inability to void but "feels the need"	Assess for length of time since the last voiding occurred
	Assess for associated symptoms such as: • Groin pain • Fever • Nausea/vomiting • Flank pain
	Suspect enlarged prostate or kidney stone

(continued)

(continued)

Finding	Action
	Encourage to seek medical attention for any new onset of symptoms
Incontinence (inability to make it to the bathroom in time)	Assess for length of time this has been occurring
	Assess for any associated symptoms
	Assess for any recent injuries or falls
	Suspect stress/urge/overflow/functional incontinence
	Encourage to seek medical attention for any new onset of symptoms
Groin pain	Assess for length of time pain has been occurring
	Assess for any associated symptoms such as: • Blood in the urine • No urine output • Flank pain
	Suspect kidney stone
	Encourage to seek medical attention for any new onset of symptoms
Drainage/bleeding from the vagina	Assess for length of time drainage/bleeding has been occurring
	Assess for last menstrual period; if postmenopausal, assess when menopause occurred
	Assess for associated symptoms such as: • Abdominal pain • Abdominal bloating • Abdominal cramping • Change in urine output, volume, and frequency

(continued)

(*continued*)

Finding	Action
	Suspect ovarian/fallopian/or uterine problem
	Encourage to seek medical attention for any new onset of symptoms
Drainage/blood from the penis	Assess for length of time drainage/bleeding has been occurring
	Assess for associated symptoms such as: • Abdominal pain • Abdominal bloating • Abdominal cramping • Change in urine output, volume, and frequency
	Suspect prostate/bladder problem
	Encourage to seek medical attention for any new onset of symptoms
Open sore on the vagina	Assess for location of the sore
	Assess for length of time sore has been present
	Assess for associated symptoms such as: • Itchiness • Vaginal drainage • Fever
	Suspect sexually transmitted infection
	Encourage to seek medical attention for any new onset of symptoms
Open sore on the penis	Assess for location of the sore
	Assess for length of time sore has been present
	Assess for associated symptoms such as: • Drainage from the penis • Swelling of the scrotum • Fever

(*continued*)

(*continued*)

Finding	Action
	Suspect sexually transmitted infection
	Encourage to seek medical attention for any new onset of symptoms
Extended erection (priapism)	Assess for length of time penis has been erect
	Assess for use of performance enhancing medication to include: ● Time of last dose ● Number of doses taken
	Assess for scrotal pain
	Suspect acute priapism
	Encourage to seek immediate medical attention
Inability to have an erection	Assess for length of time since last erection
	Assess for associated symptoms
	Assess for any changes in current medication schedule
	Suspect new onset erectile dysfunction
	Encourage to seek medical attention for any new onset of symptoms

See Chapter 18 for additional information about genitourinary system disorders.

TIPS FOR ASSESSING THE GENITOURINARY SYSTEM

● Always begin the assessment by asking if the patient/client is experiencing any problems with the body system. If not, then a general assessment would be appropriate.

- Expect hesitancy in responses when asking questions about this body system.
- This is not an assessment of sexuality or sexual practices. It focuses on current functioning and helps identify any potential or current problems.

PRACTICE EXERCISES

Read the following client situations and determine:

- Which questions to ask
- What the client might be experiencing
- If the situation is an emergency or should be followed up by a health care professional

1. During a routine care call, a client asks if it is "normal" to not "pass water" for over a day.
2. An older client says that she was told that everyone who is old loses bladder function.
3. While discussing burning with urination, a client asks if the burning caused the open sores that are all over the "private" parts.
4. While conducting a new enrollment call, a client says that the urine color is "getting better" because it used to be bright red but now it is like weak tea.
5. An older client asks if it is "normal" to have a period after not having one for over 10 years.
6. A member of a wellness program mentions having "weird" back pain that seems to "wrap around" to the lower abdomen.
7. While conducting a follow-up, postsurgical call, a client asks if is normal to feel the need to void but unable to start the stream of urine.
8. A client calls into the organization asking for suggestions with an erection that has lasted 8 hours.
9. An older client asks what can be done to "get rid of" cloudy urine.
10. A client recovering from lithotripsy says that it hurts to "pass water" because it feels like the urine is full of sand.

CASE STUDY

Oliver is reviewing the findings documented after the first call made to new enrollees in a wellness program.

- Why should Oliver make a follow-up call to these clients first?
  - Fifty-six-year-old client with osteoporosis experiencing groin pain
  - Seventy-five-year-old client recovering from prostate surgery who has not voided for 4 hours
  - Eighty-two-year-old client with perineal excoriation from incontinence

After talking with the new clients, Oliver takes an incoming call from a long-term member who is concerned about blood streaks in the urine.

- What questions should be asked first?
- What guidance should be provided to this client?

After lunch, Oliver reviews a download of new claims data for enrolled clients.

- Why should these clients be contacted for a further assessment of genitourinary function?
  - Sixty-eight-year-old client with urinalysis and complete blood count results
  - Fifty-eight-year-old client with results for an intravenous pyelogram (IVP) and kidney, ureter, and bladder (KUB) x-rays
  - Seventy-nine-year-old client with results for blood urea nitrogen (BUN), creatinine, and H & H

KEY POINTS

- The genitourinary system includes both the renal and reproductive organs.
- Not every client will need a focused assessment on this body system.

- Oftentimes, issues with the genitourinary system will be mentioned during the assessment of another body system.
- Clients may hesitate to discuss this system because of embarrassment or feeling that it is too personal to talk about.
- Approach the assessment casually and use the terms the client uses to describe symptoms.

BIBLIOGRAPHY

D'Amico, D., & Barbarito, C. (2012). *Health and physical assessment in nursing* (2nd ed.). Upper Saddle River, NJ: Pearson.

Lemone, P. (2015). *Medical-surgical nursing* (6th ed.). Upper Saddle River, NJ: Pearson.

Pearson Education. (2015). *Nursing: A concept-based approach to learning* (2nd ed., Vol. 1). Upper Saddle River, NJ: Author.

Introduction to Body System Disorders

Patients or clients are most often enrolled in a disease management program to maximize their current health status and prevent long-term complications and hospitalizations. Keep in mind, though, that not all health problems are appropriate for telephonic care.

The next chapters provide specific assessment techniques for health problems, organized by body system. Although efforts were made to be as inclusive as possible, patients may be enrolled in a program with a disease process or condition that is not represented in these pages. Should this occur, select the situations or questions that are the most appropriate to use in assessing the client and determining care needs.

CHAPTER 12

Disorders of the Integumentary System

LEARNING OUTCOMES

Upon completion of this chapter, the nurse will:

1. Summarize the different disorders of the integumentary system
2. Examine approaches to assess different disorders of the integumentary system
3. Differentiate integumentary system disorders from manifestations of systemic health problems

SKIN DISORDERS: LESIONS

Skin disorders can be divided into primary or secondary lesions. Primary lesions include:

- Cyst
- Macule or patch
- Nodule or tumor
- Papule or plaque
- Pustule
- Vesicle or bulla
- Wheal

Secondary lesions include:

- Atrophy
- Crust
- Erosion
- Fissure
- Keloid

- Lichenification
- Scales
- Scar
- Ulcer

Assessing for the presence of these lesions may be challenging when providing telephonic care; however, a great deal of information can be collected through asking focused questions.

Assessing Skin Lesions

Primary Lesion	Question
Cyst	Do you have any raised areas on the skin that feel like they are filled with fluid?
Macule or patch	Do you have any freckles or other areas on your skin that are small, round, and of a different color than the rest of your skin?
Nodule or tumor	Do you have any areas on the skin that feel hard or semisoft and seem to be deeper in the skin surface?
Papule or plaque	Do you have any skin areas that are elevated and solid like warts or moles?
Pustule	Do you have any skin areas that are oozing white–yellow colored fluid?
Vesicle or bulla	Do you have any blisters on your skin?
Wheal	Do you have any reddened areas on your skin that appear to be the result of an insect bite or hives?

Secondary Lesion	Question
Atrophy	Do you have any skin areas that appear thin, wrinkled, dry, and like tissue paper?

(*continued*)

(*continued*)

Secondary Lesion	Question
Crust	Do you have any scabs on your skin?
Erosion	Do you have any scratches on your skin?
Fissure	Do you have any cracks on the corners of your mouth or on your hands/feet?
Keloid	Do you have any scar areas that are large and raised?
Lichenification	Do you have any rough thickened areas that are rubbed consistently like on the elbows or knees?
Scales	Do you have any small pieces of flaking skin like dandruff?
Scar	Do you have any areas where the skin has healed and has left a mark?
Ulcer	Do you have any areas where the layers of the skin have been eroded?

SKIN DISORDERS: RASHES

Rashes or areas of the skin that are red and irritated can be caused by many things. The most frequent reasons for a rash include:

- Medications
- Allergies (food, chemicals, or environment)
- Systemic illness (infectious diseases)

It can be difficult to assess rashes when providing telephonic care; however, you can assess for possible causes for the disorder. When assessing, keep in mind that some rashes have distinctive patterns such as the rash associated with:

- Tinea fungal infections (round in appearance)
- Lyme disease (bull's eye appearance)
- Linear along a nerve root (herpes zoster)

Assessing Skin Rashes

Patient/Client Description	Question
If a patient relates having a rash, ask:	Where is the rash located?
	Describe the appearance
	When did the rash start?
	What have you used to treat the rash?
	Have you started any new medication?
Attempt to determine the cause:	Have you eaten anything that you normally do not eat?
	Did you receive or add any new house or outdoor plants to your environment?
	Have you gotten a new pet?
	Have you been hiking or spending time out of doors in areas where there is a large deer population?
	Have you recently slept on a bed in a hotel or other location?
	Have you recently shared towels or other personal care items with someone else?
Determine associated symptoms:	Do you have a fever?
	Did you experience an illness before the rash developed?
	Is the rash itchy? Is it itchier at different times of the day/night?
Specific reason: herpes simplex	Do you have blisters around your nose and mouth?
Specific reason: contact dermatitis	Is the rash near an area where you wear jewelry such as a ring, watch, or bracelet?
Specific reason: psoriasis	Is the rash red, raised, and thick along your elbow area and knees?
Specific reason: herpes zoster	Is the rash along the top of your chest and back? Or along the lower back/abdomen? Does the rash appear to be in a straight line?

SKIN TRAUMA

As with the skin disorders, assessing the appearance of skin trauma can be challenging. Most people describe skin trauma as "black and blue" marks; however, with careful questioning, you can help determine the extent of the trauma.

A burn is considered one of the most traumatic injuries to the skin. Although it is unlikely that a patient recovering from burn trauma will be receiving telephonic care, you might have a patient who had a previous burn injury with subsequent scarring. It would be beneficial to know where the burn occurred on the skin and the current condition of the skin surface.

Assessing Skin Trauma

Trauma	Question
"Black and blue" marks	Do you have any bruises (black and blue marks) on your body?
	Where are they located?
	Do you recall what might have caused them? Did you bump into something? Did you fall? Did something hit your skin?
	Is the tissue around the "black and blue mark" swollen or tender?
	Are the marks located just on the arms?
	Are the marks located on the abdomen?
	Are the marks located on the lower back?
	How long have the marks been there?
	Do the marks fade but are replaced with new ones?
	Are you on any medication that would thin your blood (anticoagulants, aspirin)?
	Have you discussed these marks with your (doctor, health care provider)?
Burn history	Which parts of your body were burned?
	What does the skin look like now?

(*continued*)

(*continued*)

Trauma	Question
	Would you describe your skin as puckered, thick, red, or swollen?
	Did you wear or are you still wearing a pressure garment over the burned area?

SUGGESTIONS FOR SKIN DISORDERS

- Not all patients/clients will have skin disorders. If you ask a general question about the presence of any skin lesions, rashes, or signs of trauma and the patient says "no," there is no need to go further into the assessment.
- Remember that it is impossible to determine the cause of a skin disorder with complete certainty without visually seeing the area. Be sure to relate this while talking with a patient and encourage the patient to seek medical attention for any areas that are troubling the patient.
- Depending on the type of program in which the patient is enrolled, assessment of the skin can be complicated. If the person has a systemic illness, the skin may have associated changes.
- Keep in mind that the patient/participant needs to control the conversation. If the patient is enrolled in a particular disease management program (that has absolutely nothing to do with skin disorders) and the patient is experiencing a troublesome rash or other skin condition, you should focus on that area immediately. The care or actions for the disease management program can be addressed at a later time.

PRACTICE EXERCISES

1. During the course of a telephonic conversation, the patient mentions a rash that has appeared along the lower back and extends around to the side and front of the abdomen.
   a. What questions should be asked to determine if this patient is experiencing herpes zoster?

2. A patient asks what it means when the ankles turn "black and blue."
   a. Would it be important to ask if this patient has experienced any trauma to the region?
   b. What other questions should be asked to determine the possible reason for these areas to appear?
3. A wellness call is being made. During the conversation, the participant mentions having "areas" of itchy skin. The areas are red, raised, and are located on the inner lower right leg, outer upper left thigh, upper left arm, and across the back.
   a. What do you think is the cause for these areas?
   b. What questions should you ask to obtain more information about these areas?
   c. What additional guidance should you provide to this participant?
4. An older patient with a history of lung disease and heart failure is concerned about the appearance of "black and blue" marks on both arms. The patient does not recall bumping into any furniture, and the marks just "appeared."
   a. On what should you focus when assessing for more information about these marks?

CASE STUDY

Jacquelyn, a telephonic nurse, is placing a call to Mr. Hughes, a 70-year-old patient enrolled in the cardiovascular disease management program. Currently, Mr. Hughes is recovering from hip replacement surgery. During the first call, Jacquelyn begins the assessment of the skin and learns that Mr. Hughes has:

- Swollen ankles
- "Little red marks" that just appeared on the upper chest
- Yellow drainage from the surgical site

1. What questions should Jacquelyn ask first?

   After encouraging Mr. Hughes to discuss the skin changes with the health care provider, Jacquelyn schedules another call for 5 days.

Five days later, Jacquelyn contacts Mr. Hughes who sounds irritated. Upon questioning, Mr. Hughes says:

- "I have to have some tests on my lungs because the doctor says I am having a side effect of the surgery that causes the red marks on my chest."
- "I might need more surgery because the stuff coming out of my surgery is infected."
- "I have to elevate my legs and wear those white stockings for my swollen ankles."

2. Based on these statements, what might be occurring with Mr. Hughes?

The next call was postponed because Mr. Hughes was readmitted for an incision and drainage of the total hip replacement wound site and possible treatment for other surgical complications.

3. When Mr. Hughes returns home, on what should Jacquelyn focus during the first posthospital assessment?

KEY POINTS

- Skin disorders can occur in isolation or be related to another health problem.
- If the patient says that there are no problems with the skin, do not continue with a specific assessment.
- If the patient mentions the onset or presence of a skin disorder, take the time to further assess the condition even if that is not the primary purpose of the call.
- Encourage the patient to seek medical attention for any skin condition or changes that do not appear to be healing, are becoming worse, or are troubling to the patient.

BIBLIOGRAPHY

D'Amico, D., & Barbarito, C. (2012). *Health and physical assessment in nursing* (2nd ed.). Upper Saddle River, NJ: Pearson.
Lemone, P. (2015). *Medical-surgical nursing* (6th ed.). Upper Saddle River, NJ: Pearson.

CHAPTER 13

Disorders of the Respiratory System

LEARNING OUTCOMES

Upon completion of this chapter, the nurse will:

1. Summarize the different disorders of the respiratory system
2. Examine approaches to assess different disorders of the respiratory system
3. Determine approaches that can be used for more than one respiratory disorder

RESPIRATORY DISORDERS

The respiratory disorders can be divided into those that affect the upper respiratory or lower respiratory tracts. The major disorders of the upper respiratory tract include:

- Common cold
- Influenza
- Sinusitis
- Pharyngitis
- Laryngeal cancer
- Sleep apnea

And the major disorders of the lower respiratory tract are:

- Asthma
- Bronchitis
- Pneumonia

- Emphysema
- Chronic obstructive lung/pulmonary disease (COLD/COPD)
- Tuberculosis
- Lung cancer

Assessing the patient/client with these respiratory disorders may be challenging mainly because the client could be experiencing shortness of breath. Although open-ended questions are encouraged during the telephonic assessment, closed-ended questions might be easier for the client to answer. Carefully listen to the client's breathing and speech pattern when beginning a call to a client with a known respiratory disorder. If the client is having difficulty in breathing and talking, change the questions to closed-ended or consider rescheduling the call to when the client's breathing has stabilized or improved.

ASSESSING UPPER RESPIRATORY CONDITIONS

Health Problem	Question
Common cold	Are you experiencing nasal stuffiness, sneezing, watery eyes, and a scratchy throat?
	How would you describe what you are experiencing?
	What have you been doing to treat the symptoms?
	Has the treatment been effective?
Influenza	Are you experiencing body aches/pains, tiredness, nasal stuffiness, and a raspy cough?
	Did you receive a flu vaccination this season?
	How long have you been feeling this way?
	What are you doing to help with the symptoms?
Sinusitis	How long has your voice sounded nasal?
	Has this ever happened to you before?
	Are you feeling any fullness of pressure along your forehead or alongside your nose and cheekbones?
	Does your head feel full when you lean forward?
	What are you doing to help with the symptoms?

(continued)

(continued)

Health Problem	Question
Pharyngitis	How long has your voice sounded hoarse or raspy?
	Is your throat sore?
	Are you able to drink fluids?
	Have you taken your temperature? • If so, what was your last temperature?
	What are you doing to help with the symptoms?
Laryngeal cancer	(For telephonic care, the client with a history of laryngeal cancer will most likely use a device to assist with verbal communication. The sound of the device is very distinctive and sounds mechanical. Talking with these clients is not tiring or painful but ask if the client feels up to carrying on a conversation before proceeding.) It sounds like you are using something to help you talk. Can you tell me what you are using and why?
	When were you diagnosed with laryngeal cancer?
	Are you still undergoing treatment?
	Are you experiencing any other symptoms because of it?
Sleep apnea	Have you ever had a test where you slept in a laboratory overnight and your breathing was measured?
	Have you ever been told that you stop breathing while you are asleep?
	Do you use a machine at home to keep your airway open when you sleep?
	Do you place the device in your nose or your mouth?
	Do you use the device every night?
	Are you having any difficulty or issues with using the device?

ASSESSING LOWER RESPIRATORY CONDITIONS

It is likely that clients with a lower respiratory condition will be enrolled in a disease management program. Even so, it is important for you to assess the client's current status and if any new manifestations are occurring. Keep in mind that the client may be short of breath or fatigued. The episodes of telephonic care may be shorter but more frequently conducted. Consider the following techniques when assessing a client with any of these lower respiratory conditions:

Health Problem	Question
Asthma	When were you diagnosed with asthma?
	What do you avoid so that you don't experience an asthma attack? (document as triggers)
	When was your most recent asthma attack?
	How often do you have acute attacks?
	Describe what happens to you when you have an asthma attack. ● Does your chest become tight? ● Do you start to wheeze or make noises when you breathe? ● Do you become short of breath?
	Have you ever been hospitalized because of your asthma?
	Do you have a peak flow meter at home?
	Do you use the peak flow meter? ● If so, what was your last "color"? (Peak flow meter readings are estimated according to traffic signal colors: Green indicates asthma is under control; yellow means asthma is somewhat controlled; red means the client needs immediate medical attention.)
	What medications do you take to control the asthma?

(*continued*)

(continued)

Health Problem	Question
	Do you take any of these medications as an inhaler? ● Is the inhaler meter-dosed or dry powder?
	How often do you use a rescue bronchodilator inhaler during the day?
	How often do you see your doctor or health care provider for the asthma?
Bronchitis	How often do you experience episodes of bronchitis?
	Are you coughing up phlegm? ● What color is the phlegm?
	Are you experiencing any pain when you cough? ● Where is the pain located?
	What causes the bronchitis to occur? ● Smoking? ● Environmental irritants?
	What do you do to reduce the symptoms of bronchitis?
	What medications are you prescribed for the bronchitis?
	How often do you see your doctor or health care provider for the bronchitis?
Pneumonia	Did your doctor or health care provider tell you what type of pneumonia you have?
	How often do you experience episodes of pneumonia?
	Have you received the pneumonia vaccination? ● When did you receive it?
	What are your current symptoms? ● Cough? ● Phlegm production and color? ● Chest pain with coughing? ● Fatigue/sleepiness?
	What medication have you been prescribed for the pneumonia? ● Has the medication been helping?

(continued)

(*continued*)

Health Problem	Question
	What else have you been doing to help with the pneumonia? ◦ Increasing oral fluids? ◦ Getting more rest? ◦ Not smoking/avoiding cigarette smoke?
Emphysema/COPD	When were you diagnosed with emphysema/COPD?
	Did you or are you currently smoking cigarettes? ◦ When did you start smoking cigarettes? ◦ How many packs of cigarettes do you smoke each day? ◦ Have you tried to stop smoking cigarettes? ◦ Are you interested in smoking cessation information?
	What symptoms do you experience on a daily basis? ◦ Cough? ◦ Phlegm production? Color, consistency, and amount? ◦ Pain with coughing? ◦ Shortness of breath?
	What is your activity level right now? ◦ Do you become short of breath when walking short distances? ◦ Are you able to complete your own basic care such as bathing, dressing, and going to the bathroom? ◦ Are you able to shop and prepare your own meals? ◦ How many times do you need to stop, sit, and catch your breath when engaging in activities?
	Do you wear oxygen? (portable oxygen concentrator) ◦ Do you wear it continuously? ◦ Do you have an oxygen concentrator in the home? ◦ What is the setting for your oxygen (liters per minute)? ◦ Do you use a face mask or the prongs in the nose (nasal cannula)?
	How often do you develop or experience lung infections?

(*continued*)

(*continued*)

Health Problem	Question
	What is your current weight? ● Have you lost/gained weight over the last few months?
	How would you rate your appetite (poor, fair, or good)? ● Has your appetite changed over the last few months? ● Do you experience shortness of breath when eating?
	How much fluid do you drink each day? ● Have you been instructed to increase/decrease fluid intake by your doctor or health care provider?
	What medication have you been prescribed for the emphysema/COPD? ● Has your breathing improved with the medication?
	What else have you been doing to help with your breathing?
	Have you been instructed in any coughing techniques to help clear your lungs? ● Pursed lip breathing? ● Diaphragmatic breathing? ● Huff coughing?
	How often do you see your doctor/health care provider for your breathing?
Tuberculosis	When were you diagnosed with tuberculosis?
	What were your symptoms? ● Cough with bloody phlegm? ● Weight loss? ● Fatigue? ● Night sweating?
	What testing did you have done? ● Skin test? ● Chest x-ray? ● Sputum samples?
	What medication have you been prescribed? ● Are you taking the medication as prescribed? Why or why not?

(*continued*)

(continued)

Health Problem	Question
	Are you experiencing any "odd" effects from the medication? ● Change in urine/feces/tears/sweat color? (Rifampin can change body fluids to orange-red in color) ● Tingling of the hands or feet? (Isoniazid would be prescribed to prevent this) ● Changes in seeing colors in your vision? (Ethambutol can affect red-green color discrimination and visual acuity) ● Changes in hearing? (Streptomycin is ototoxic and affects hearing)
	How long have you been told that you need to take this medication?
	How are you feeling right now? ● Improved appetite? ● Weight gain? ● Less night sweats? ● Reduced coughing? ● Color of phlegm improved?
	How often do you see your doctor/health care provider? ● When is your next appointment? ● When was your last sputum sample?
Lung cancer	A patient with a diagnosis of lung cancer might be enrolled in another disease management program. It is rare for a disease management program to be created for an oncological health problem. General questions appropriate for this health problem are as follows:
	When were you diagnosed with the lung cancer?
	What treatment have you or are you receiving for the problem? ● Chemotherapy? ● Radiation? ● Surgery?
	How are you feeling right now?
	Are you experiencing any shortness of breath?

(continued)

(*continued*)

Health Problem	Question
	Are you experiencing any effects from the treatment? ● Poor appetite? ● Weight loss? ● Mouth sores? ● Fatigue/sleepiness?
	How often do you have a treatment?
	How long will you be getting treatments?
	Are you able to: ● Perform self-care? Bathing, toileting, dressing? ● Shop and prepare meals for yourself?
	Are you wearing or using oxygen? ● Is it continuous or only when you feel short of breath? ● Do you have a portable oxygen container to use when you go out of doors? ● Do you have an oxygen concentrator in the home? ● Do you use a face mask or nasal prongs for the oxygen?
	Are you experiencing any pain? ● Where is the pain? ● How would you rate the pain on a scale from 1 to 10 with 1 being no or minimal pain to 10 being the worst possible pain? ● What helps with the pain? ● How often do you take pain medication if prescribed?
	What other medications have you been prescribed for your lung cancer?
	When is your next doctor/health care provider appointment?

SUGGESTIONS FOR RESPIRATORY DISORDERS

● Clients may be hesitant to admit of a chronic health problem. This could be due to the fear of losing health insurance coverage or having this information shared with an employer. Ensure the client that all information collected is confidential and not reported back to the health plan or employer.

- Clients may be frustrated with having a respiratory problem and sound annoyed with the questioning. Keep in mind that the client may be short of breath. Do not keep the client on the telephone for extended periods of time. Structure more assessment questions to have yes/no answers (closed-ended). Offer the client guidance, encouragement, and support.

- Clients may have a chronic cough caused by smoking. Oftentimes the client would have already been counselled about smoking cessation and may not want to hear anything more about it. The only way to know how the client will respond is to ask. If the client becomes angry, do not insist on smoking cessation at this time. If the client acknowledges that smoking is contributing/ causing the health problem, proceed with discussing options for smoking cessation. There is no major potion for smoking cessation. Most individuals who have successfully stopped smoking tried a variety of techniques and cessation aides such as nicotine patches or chewing gum and support groups. The client may be encouraged to discuss smoking cessation actions with the doctor/health care provider who may prescribe medication to assist in the process.

- Clients may have a diagnosis of chronic lung disease and use oxygen periodically in the home. During the course of a conversation, you may learn that the client continues to smoke cigarettes. Be sure to emphasize that smoking should not be done in the home with an oxygen concentrator. Emphasize that this is a fire hazard. Follow up in a few days with another telephone call to reinforce the information about oxygen safety.

- Clients being treated for lung cancer may convey depression about the diagnosis and prognosis. Realize that these conversations and episodes of care provide the client with opportunities to discuss thoughts, feelings, and reactions to treatment. Do not approach these calls as being futile because the client is terminally ill. Provide as much emotional and caring support as possible.

- Clients may have limited financial resources and be unable to afford medications prescribed for asthma. Take the time to explain or reinforce actions to reduce the risk of asthma attacks.

Brainstorm ways for the client to be able to find resources to pay for the needed medication. Suggest that the client discuss the financial hardship with the doctor/health care provider who may be able to prescribe a less costly medication or have access to pharmaceutical representatives who could have coupons or samples that can be shared with the client.

• Clients with tuberculosis may admit to stopping their medication because of adverse effects. Gently remind the client that the health problem is treatable and is not chronic. Ask if the adverse effects have been discussed with the doctor/health care provider. The medications may need to be altered or changed, which would reduce or eliminate the adverse effects while continuing to treat the infection.

PRACTICE EXERCISES

1. During the course of a conversation you learn that a client has been coughing blood for several weeks and has not scheduled an appointment to see the doctor/health care provider.
   a. What additional questions should you ask this client?
   b. What should you say to the client in response to the decision to not seek medical attention?
2. A client with COPD expresses anger with himself about smoking for so many years. The client now needs to continuously wear oxygen and is unable to provide self-care activities.
   a. What should you say to encourage this client?
   b. What suggestions could you make to help improve the client's stamina and energy level?
3. A client who has been experiencing weight loss, night sweats, and "dark" flecks of material in the sputum had a "shot placed on the inside of the arm" a few days ago. The area became very red, swollen, and itchy; however, the client never returned to the doctor/health care provider to have the area assessed.
   a. What would be a priority for this client?
   b. What should you suggest that the client do immediately after ending the telephone call?

4. A client with a known history of asthma has been changing the frequency and amount of prescribed medications because of being "tired" of having to constantly use inhalers and take pills.
   a. What would be important for you to emphasize with this client?
   b. What can you do with the client over the phone to determine the client's current lung/breathing status?

CASE STUDY

You receive a list of new clients to contact because of recent enrollment in a respiratory disease management program. While beginning to explain the program on the first call, the client hangs up the telephone.

- What would you do?
- What would you document in the client's record?

The next client has a history of chronic lung disease and sounds "out of breath" when answering the telephone.

- What questions would be the most important for you to ask on this first call?
- How would you know if the client is having difficulty in talking?

Before lunch, you decide to place one more call to a client with a history of asthma. When the call is answered, you learn that the client has just returned from jogging through the neighborhood and has audible wheezes.

- What direction should you provide to the client?
- Once the client's breathing improves, what guidance should you offer to reduce the risk of another acute asthma attack after exercising?

KEY POINTS

- Listen carefully to how the patient/client talks and breathes over the telephone.
- Keep questions brief.

- Focus assessment questions based on the information you have or learned while on the call with the patient/client.
- Keep the length of the call to a minimum. Reschedule for another call within a few days.
- Be aware of all patients/clients who have home oxygen. Reinforce home safety with an oxygen concentrator on every call.

BIBLIOGRAPHY

D'Amico, D., & Barbarito, C. (2012). *Health and physical assessment in nursing* (2nd ed.). Upper Saddle River, NJ: Pearson.

Lemone, P. (2015). *Medical-surgical nursing* (6th ed.). Upper Saddle River, NJ: Pearson.

CHAPTER 14

Disorders of the Cardiovascular System

LEARNING OUTCOMES

Upon completion of this chapter, the nurse will:

1. Summarize the different disorders of the cardiovascular system
2. Examine approaches to assess different disorders of the cardiovascular system
3. Determine approaches that can be used for more than one cardiovascular disorder

CARDIOVASCULAR DISORDERS

The cardiovascular disorders can be categorized according to the structures affected. The cardiac disorders listed would be the ones most commonly identified for disease management telephonic care. Some cardiac disorders require hospitalization for treatment, such as disseminating intravascular coagulation and sudden cardiac death, and would not be appropriate for telephonic care.

For the heart, these disorders would be:

- Myocardial infarction
- Angina
- Dysrhythmias
- Heart failure
- Valvular dysfunction
- Endocarditis
- Coronary artery disease

For the arterial system, these disorders include:

- Atherosclerosis
- Peripheral arterial disease

- Hypertension
- Aneurysms

Disorders associated with the venous system include:

- Peripheral venous disease
- Varicose veins
- Deep vein thrombosis

For the lymphatic system, the client might experience:

- Lymphedema
- Enlarged/swollen lymph glands

Disorders associated or that affect the blood system include:

- Anemia
- Sickle cell disease
- Leukemia
- Lymphoma
- Hemophilia

ASSESSING DISORDERS OF THE HEART

Remember that the client is already diagnosed with a heart problem. When providing telephonic care, you are assessing the client's current condition, symptoms, and if anything has changed or needs to be referred to the doctor/health care professional.

Health Problem	Question
Recovering from an acute myocardial infarction	How are you feeling right now?
	Are you experiencing any chest pain similar to the pain that you had when you had your "heart attack?"
	How is your energy level?
	How much sleep are you getting each night?
	How many rest periods (and for how long) are you taking each day?
	Are you scheduled to attend cardiac rehabilitation? When do you attend?

(continued)

(continued)

Health Problem	Question
	Are you taking all of your medications as prescribed? ● Do you have any questions about the medications, the expected effects, or any side effects that you might be experiencing?
	Have you been told when you can: ● Return to work? ● Resume normal activity?
	Have you been prescribed a special diet to follow? ● Do you have any questions about the diet?
History of angina	Describe the type of chest pain that you usually experience
	What are you supposed to do when you have the chest pain? ● Are you following what you are supposed to do when you have the chest pain?
	Do you have a bottle of nitroglycerin tablets to use?
	Are the pills in the original bottle from the pharmacy?
	Have you had the nitroglycerin pills replaced within the last 6 months?
	For what reasons have you been directed by your doctor or health care provider to seek additional medical care when you are having the chest pain?
Diagnosed with an atrial dysrhythmia	What medication are you taking for the dysrhythmia?
	Do you have to have your blood drawn periodically?
	Does your medication dose change after having your blood drawn?
	Are you experiencing any bleeding or bruising since starting to take the medication for the dysrhythmia?

(continued)

(continued)

Health Problem	Question
	Did you have or are you scheduled to have any surgery or procedures to correct the dysrhythmia? • When did you have the procedure/when is the procedure scheduled?
	Do you have a pacemaker? • When was it inserted? • When was it last checked? • When was the battery last changed?
	For what reasons have you been directed by your doctor/health care provider to seek additional medical care because of the dysrhythmia?
Diagnosed with a ventricular dysrhythmia	What medication are you taking for the dysrhythmia?
	Did you have or are you scheduled to have any surgery or procedures to correct the dysrhythmia? • What did you have done/what are you scheduled to have done? • When did you have the procedure done/when are you scheduled to have the procedure done?
	Do you have a pacemaker? • When was it inserted? • When was it last checked? • When was the battery last changed?
	Do you have something called an implanted defibrillator? • Has it ever gone off? • What did it feel like when it went off? • Have you been directed to do anything in particular when it goes off?
	For what reasons have you been directed by your doctor or health care provider to seek additional medical care because of the dysrhythmia?
Diagnosed with heart failure	How are you feeling right now?

(continued)

(continued)

Health Problem	Question
	What medications are you taking for your heart problem?
	Are you routinely coughing? • Is the cough new, since starting any medication? • Are you producing any phlegm? • What color is the phlegm?
	Are you having any problems catching your breath?
	Do you wear oxygen? • All the time or only when short of breath? • Do you have an oxygen concentrator in the home? • Do you have a portable oxygen unit to use when you go out?
	Are you having any swelling of the feet/ankles/lower legs?
	Do your shoes feel tight?
	Are your rings tight on your fingers?
	For what reasons have you been directed by your doctor or health care provider to seek additional medical care because of the heart problem?
Valvular dysfunction	When were you told you had a problem with a valve in your heart?
	Are you scheduled for surgery?
	Did you have valve replacement surgery? • Would you know what kind of valve was used as a replacement? • Can you hear a click through your chest? (Mechanical valves will click. Bovine or porcine valves will not click.)
	Are you taking any medication after having the valve replaced? (Mechanical valves will need lifetime anticoagulation. Bovine/porcine valves will not need any anticoagulation.)

(continued)

(continued)

Health Problem	Question
	For what reasons have you been directed by your doctor or health care provider to seek additional medical care because of the valve problem?
Endocarditis	How are you feeling right now?
	Were you told the reason for your heart infection?
	Are you taking any medication right now for the infection? • How long do you have to take it?
	Have you been directed to avoid any activities because of the heart infection?
	Have you been directed to change your diet because of the heart infection?
	Have you been directed to change your lifestyle because of the heart infection? (Endocarditis has been associated with substance abuse.)
	For what reasons have you been directed by your doctor/health care provider to seek additional medical care because of the heart infection?
Coronary artery disease	How are you feeling right now?
	What have you been told about the blockages in your heart vessels?
	Have you had a procedure or surgery to place something called a stent in your heart vessels? • When was this done?
	Are you taking any medication since the stents were placed?
	Are you scheduled or planning to have the vessels replaced?/Have you had the vessels replaced? • When will this be done?/When was this done?
	Are you on any new medication since the vessels were replaced?

(continued)

(*continued*)

Health Problem	Question
	Have you been directed to change your diet since the vessels were replaced?
	Have you had to alter your activity status since the vessels were replaced?
	Have you had to make lifestyle changes since the vessels were replaced? (Modifiable risk factors for coronary artery disease include weight reduction, exercise, smoking cessation, low-fat diet, low-sodium diet.)
	For what reasons have you been directed by your doctor/health care provider to seek additional medical care because of the heart vessels?

ASSESSING DISORDERS OF THE ARTERIAL SYSTEM

Health Problem	Question
Diagnosed with atherosclerosis/ peripheral arterial disease	How are you feeling right now?
	Do you have pain in your calves (back of your lower legs) when you walk?
	Do your legs ache when sitting down?
	Do you have numbness or tingling in your legs and feet?
	Do the fronts of your lower legs look red when your feet are flat on the floor?
	Do you smoke cigarettes? ● When did you start smoking? ● How much do you smoke each day? ● Have you considered stopping smoking? (Smoking is a modifiable risk factor for the development of atherosclerosis.)

(*continued*)

(continued)

Health Problem	Question
	Have you been directed to make any changes because of the atherosclerosis such as: • A low-fat diet? • Increasing activity/walking? • Reducing body weight?
	Are you taking or have been prescribed medications for the atherosclerosis?
	For what reasons have you been directed by your doctor or health care provider to seek additional medical care because of the atherosclerosis?
Hypertension	How are you feeling right now?
	Do you know what your last blood pressure measurement was?
	What medications have you been prescribed for the high blood pressure? • Are you taking the medication as directed? • Are you experiencing any other effects from the medication?
	Have you been directed to make any other changes to help reduce your blood pressure such as: • Weight reduction? • Increase activity/exercise? • Smoking cessation? • Low sodium diet (dietary approaches to stop hypertension [DASH] diet)? • Stress management? • Reduce alcohol intake?
	For what reasons have you been directed by your doctor or health care provider to seek additional medical care because of the high blood pressure?
Diagnosed with or recovering from treatment for an aneurysm	How are you feeling right now?
	Where is/was your aneurysm located?

(continued)

(continued)

Health Problem	Question
	How was it/is it going to be treated? • What type of surgery did you have/are scheduled to have? • When did you have/are scheduled to have the surgery?
	Are you taking or prescribed any medications for the aneurysm (vessel weakness)? • How often do you take this medication? • Has your doctor/health care provider told you how long you will need to take the medication?
	Have you been directed to make lifestyle changes such as: • Smoking cessation? • Weight reduction? • Dietary changes? • Measures to prevent constipation/straining at a stool? • Avoiding prolonged sitting, lifting heavy objects, strenuous exercise?
	For what reasons have you been directed by your doctor/health care provider to seek additional medical care because of the aneurysm (vessel weakness)?

ASSESSING DISORDERS OF THE VENOUS SYSTEM

Health Problem	Question
Peripheral venous/ vascular disease	How are you feeling right not?
	Do your lower legs ever feel itchy?
	Do your lower legs swell more after standing for long periods of time?
	Do your legs ever start to hurt when standing?

(continued)

(continued)

Health Problem	Question
	What color is your skin over the front of your lower legs? (Cyanosis and brown pigmentation of the lower leg and feet are associated with peripheral vascular disease [PVD]).
	Are there any areas of fluid leaking through the tissue on the front of your lower legs?
	Do you have any open sores around your ankles?
	Have you been directed to wear compression stockings?
	Have you been directed to elevate your feet and legs throughout the day?
	Do you smoke cigarettes? ● When did you start smoking? ● How much do you smoke each day? ● Have you considered stopping smoking? (Smoking is a modifiable risk factor for the development of PVD.)
	Have you been directed to make any changes because of your veins such as: ● A low-fat diet? ● Increasing activity/walking? ● Reducing body weight?
	Are you taking or have been prescribed medications for your veins?
	For what reasons have you been directed by your doctor/health care provider to seek additional medical care because of the veins?
Varicose veins	How are your legs feeling right now?
	Do your legs feel: ● Heavy? ● Fatigued/tired? ● Aching? ● Warm or hot?

(continued)

(*continued*)

Health Problem	Question
	Have you been directed to make any lifestyle changes such as: • Smoking cessation? • Weight reduction?
	What treatment have you been prescribed for the varicose veins such as: • Wearing compression stockings? • Frequently elevating your legs? • Increasing walking every day? • Avoiding prolonged standing/sitting?
	Have you been prescribed any medication to treat the varicose veins?
	Are you considering/scheduled for surgery to treat the varicose veins? • When is the surgery scheduled/was the surgery?
	For what reasons have you been directed by your doctor/health care provider to seek additional medical care because of the varicose veins?
Deep vein thrombosis	How are you feeling right now?
	Which leg/body part was affected by the blood clot?
	What medication have you been taking for the blood clot? • Do you have to have your blood checked periodically because of the medication? • How long have you been told that you will need to take the medication?
	Have you been directed to make any lifestyle changes because of the blood clot?
	Have you been directed to avoid performing any activities because of the blood clot?
	For what reasons have you been directed by your doctor/health care provider to seek additional medical care because of the blood clot?

ASSESSING DISORDERS OF THE LYMPHATIC SYSTEM

Health Problem	Question
Diagnosed with lymphedema	Which body area is swollen/edematous?
	Have you been told the reason why the body area is swollen?
	What treatment have you been prescribed for the swelling such as: ● Elevating the limb? ● Wearing compression stockings?
	Have you been directed to avoid any activities because of the swelling?
	Have you been prescribed any medication for the swelling?
	For what reasons have you been directed by your doctor or health care provider to seek additional medical care because of the swelling?
Enlarged/swollen lymph glands	Where are the swollen lymph glands/nodes located?
	Have you been told why the lymph nodes have become swollen?
	Are the swellings painful?
	What are you doing to control the pain? ● Have you been prescribed medication for the pain?
	Have you been prescribed any medication to treat the swelling? ● Is the medication helping reduce the swelling?
	For what reasons have you been directed by your doctor or health care provider to seek additional medical care because of the swollen lymph nodes?

ASSESSING DISORDERS OF THE BLOOD SYSTEM

Health Problem	Question
Anemia	What type/kind of anemia do you have?
	How are you feeling right now?
	What symptoms are you experiencing because of the anemia? ● Iron deficiency: brittle, spoon-shaped nails, cracks at the corners of the mouth, sore tongue, craving unusual items to eat? ● Vitamin B_{12} deficiency: paleness, weakness, sore red tongue, diarrhea, numbness, and tingling of the hands and feet? ● Folic acid deficiency: weakness and fatigue, paleness, shortness of breath, heart palpitations?
	What have you been prescribed to treat the anemia? ● Oral supplement/replacements? ● Dietary changes? ● Reduce alcohol intake?
	Have the treatments improved how you feel?
	For what reasons have you been directed by your doctor or health care provider to seek additional medical care because of the anemia?
Sickle cell anemia	When were you first told that you have sickle cell anemia?
	How are you feeling right now?
	Have you had to be hospitalized for a crisis?
	What medications have you been prescribed for the anemia?
	Have you been directed to: ● Increase fluids? ● Get extra rest? ● Avoid stress?
	For what reasons have you been directed by your doctor or health care provider to seek additional medical care because of the anemia?

(*continued*)

(*continued*)

Health Problem	Question
Leukemia	What type of blood problem do you have? (Some clients may not want to say leukemia but call it something else such as "not enough white blood cells" or "a disease that causes me to be weak.")
	How long have you had this blood problem?
	What type of treatment are you receiving for the blood problem? ● Chemotherapy? ● Radiation? ● Scheduled for a bone marrow transplant? ● Stem cell transplant?
	How are you feeling right now?
	What have you been directed to do to help improve your health? ● Avoid crowds? ● Practice good handwashing technique? ● Thoroughly wash fresh fruits and vegetables? ● Increase protein/calorie intake by eating small frequent meals? ● Use a soft toothbrush? ● Avoid strenuous activity or exercise? ● Use a bulk-forming laxative? ● Avoid all sharp objects?
	For what reasons have you been directed by your doctor/health care provider to seek additional medical care because of the blood problem?
Lymphoma	What was used to diagnose your health problem? ● A swollen gland that would not heal? ● Fever? ● Night sweats? ● Fatigue? ● Weight loss? ● Abdominal pain? ● Nausea? ● Vomiting? ● Headaches?
	How are you feeling right now?

(*continued*)

(*continued*)

Health Problem	Question
	What is being done to treat your health problem? ● Chemotherapy? ● Radiation? ● Stem cell transplant?
	What have you been directed to do to help improve your health? ● Special skin care? ● Increase rest periods? ● Actions to reduce/prevent nausea? ● Increase protein/calorie intake with small frequent meals? ● Avoid strenuous activity or exercise?
	For what reasons have you been directed by your doctor/health care provider to seek additional medical care because of the health problem?
Hemophilia	When were you first told you had a problem with your blood clotting?
	What are your usual symptoms? ● Bruising? ● Swollen knees? ● Bleeding gums? ● Blood in your stool? ● Vomiting blood? ● Nosebleeds?
	What medications are you prescribed for the blood clotting problem?
	How are you feeling right now?
	What have you been directed to do to help prevent bleeding? ● Avoid medications with aspirin? ● Avoid sharp objects? ● Use electric razor? ● Wear a medical alert bracelet or neck tag? ● Practice gentle oral hygiene?
	For what reasons have you been directed by your doctor/health care provider to seek additional medical care because of the blood clotting problem?

SUGGESTIONS FOR CARDIOVASCULAR DISORDERS

- Find out the term or words the client uses to describe the problem. Some clients may not want to say "heart failure" or "cancer."
- Ask first how the client is currently feeling with the health problem. Usual symptoms can be assessed afterward.
- Determine if the client is prescribed any specific medication or treatment for the health problem. Ask if the client has been adhering to what has been prescribed and if the treatment or medication has helped. If the client is not adhering to the prescribed treatment or medication, find out why. Brainstorm ways with the client to help improve adherence if possible.
- Reinforce prescribed treatment or therapy. Do not suggest alternative treatment approaches.
- Once the acute/chronic cardiovascular problem has been assessed, find out if the client is experiencing any other issues that may need to be addressed.
- Take the client's lead when contacting the client about a chronic cardiovascular problem. The client may not want to spend time talking about it.
- Be sure to give the client sufficient time to discuss the problem, medications, treatments, or any other therapy to enhance wellness.

PRACTICE EXERCISES

Read the following client situations and determine:

- Which questions to ask
- What the client might be experiencing
- Whether the situation requires the client to contact the doctor or health care provider

1. An older client recovering from pacemaker insertion for an atrial dysrhythmia is experiencing slurred speech and confusion while talking on the telephone.
2. A client who is prescribed methadone was recently discharged from the hospital for treatment of endocarditis.
3. A client with an elevated cholesterol level notices that both feet are swelling and a small open area has developed on the right inner ankle.

4. A client who works as a hairdresser is experiencing leg heaviness and itching after standing for several hours at work.
5. A client with a history of hemophilia has been experiencing right knee pain. The skin is warm to touch and "blown up like a balloon."
6. A client with lymphoma asks if "it's ok" to use a cleanser to "scrub off the marks" that were made on his skin for the radiation treatments.

CASE STUDY

Quincy has been providing telephonic care for a disease management program for several years. When the phone is answered, Quincy notices that the client sounds out of breath. When asked about the breathing, the client states that she had to walk to the other room to get the telephone. After sitting for a few minutes, the client's breathing becomes normal.

- Which cardiovascular health problems can cause shortness of breath?
- What additional information should be asked to determine if the client has a cardiovascular problem?

Quincy learns that the client had an acute myocardial infarction a month ago and is being treated for iron deficiency anemia. The client asks if it is "normal" for the stool to look "black."

- What information about the client's treatment is needed before responding to the client's question?
- What other information about the client's bowel movements would be important to assess?

Overall, the client says that she is feeling "pretty good" considering that she had a heart attack a month ago and asks when she can have a cigarette.

- How should this question be answered?
- What information about smoking cessation should be shared with the client?

Quincy learns that the client has been prescribed cardiac rehabilitation but missed the last session because of "feeling tired."

The client asks how long the rehabilitation was going to last because she wanted to return to work and not feel like an invalid.

- How should you respond to the client skipping cardiac rehabilitation?
- What can you say to encourage the client to attend the sessions?
- What words of encouragement can you provide to reduce the client feeling like an invalid?

Quincy schedules a follow-up call to be made in 5 days.

- What should be the focus of the next call?
- What additional information may need to be prepared prior to the next call?

KEY POINTS

- There are many disorders that affect the cardiovascular system.
- Most clients are aware of having a cardiac disorder.
- Use the clients' terminology when discussing the disorder.
- Be aware of the client's behavior during the call. If recently discharged from the hospital, the client may feel fatigued and not want to talk for long periods of time.
- At all times, reinforce the prescribed treatment for the health problem. Refer the client to contact the doctor/health care provider with any specific questions.

BIBLIOGRAPHY

American Heart Association. (n.d.). Atherosclerosis. Retrieved from http://www.heart.org/HEARTORG/Conditions/Cholesterol/WhyCholesterolMatters/Atherosclerosis_UCM_305564_Article.jsp#.Vzrvdr7Au31

D'Amico, D., & Barbarito, C. (2012). *Health and physical assessment in nursing* (2nd ed.). Upper Saddle River, NJ: Pearson.

Lemone, P. (2015). *Medical-surgical nursing* (6th ed.). Upper Saddle River, NJ: Pearson.

Pearson Education. (2015). *Nursing: A concept-based approach to learning* (2nd ed., Vol. 2). Upper Saddle River, NJ: Author.

CHAPTER 15

Disorders of the Gastrointestinal System

LEARNING OUTCOMES

Upon completion of this chapter, the nurse will:

1. Summarize the different disorders of the gastrointestinal system
2. Examine approaches to assess different disorders of the gastrointestinal system
3. Determine approaches that can be used for more than one gastrointestinal disorder

GASTROINTESTINAL DISORDERS

Disorders of the gastrointestinal system can be categorized according to the body area or organ affected. The disorders identified are the most common ones appropriate for telephonic care and include:

- Stomatitis
- Gastroesophageal reflux disease (GERD)
- Gastric ulcers/duodenal ulcers
- Small bowel obstruction
- Crohn's disease
- Ulcerative colitis
- Irritable bowel syndrome
- Diverticulitis/diverticulosis
- Appendicitis
- Liver cirrhosis
- Hepatitis
- Cholelithiasis
- Cholecystitis

- Acute pancreatitis
- Chronic pancreatitis
- Eating disorders
  - Anorexia nervosa
  - Bulimia nervosa

ASSESSING DISORDERS OF THE GASTROINTESTINAL SYSTEM

Remember that the client is already diagnosed with a gastrointestinal problem. When providing telephonic care, you are assessing the client's current condition, symptoms, and if anything has changed or needs to be referred to the health care professional.

Health Problem	Question
Stomatitis	When did you start having mouth ulcers?
	What was the reason they developed? ● Were they related to poorly fitting dentures or other dental prostheses?
	How are the ulcers right now?
	Are you using any specific medicine for them? If so, ● What is the name of the medicine? ● How often do you use it?
	Do the ulcers cause you much pain? If so, ● What do you do for the pain?
	Have you changed your diet because of the ulcers? If so, ● What foods do you avoid? ● What foods are you able to tolerate?
	Have you gained/lost weight because of the mouth ulcers?

(continued)

(continued)

Health Problem	Question
	For what reasons have you been directed by your doctor or health care provider to seek additional medical care because of the mouth ulcers?
GERD	When were you diagnosed with GERD?
	What were you told was the reason that it developed?
	What symptoms do you experience when the GERD is "acting up"? Such as, • Burping up food from the stomach? • Chest pain? • Sore throat? • Hoarseness? • Belching? • Problems swallowing? • Pain when eating? • Chronic cough?
	What causes the symptoms? For example, • Food? • Alcohol intake? • Stress? • Bending over after eating? • Lying down flat in bed?
	Have you been avoiding certain foods because of it? Such as foods that are: • Acidic? • Fatty? • Spicy?
	What medicine are you taking for the GERD? • How long have you been instructed to take it? • Does it help with the symptoms?

(continued)

(continued)

Health Problem	Question
	What else have you been instructed to do to help with the GERD, such as: • Smoking cessation? • Avoid wearing tight clothing? • Maintain body weight or lose weight? • Eat smaller more frequent meals? • Avoid eating for several hours before going to bed? • Staying upright for several hours after eating? • Elevating the head of the bed on blocks?
	For what reasons have you been directed by your doctor or health care provider to seek additional medical care because of the GERD?
Gastric/duodenal ulcers	When were you told that you had a gastric/duodenal ulcer?
	What were/are your symptoms? Such as: • Pain (describe the pain; some common terms include gnawing, aching, or extreme hunger)? ▪ Does eating make the pain go away? • Heartburn? • Vomiting coffee-ground appearing material?
	Are you taking an antibiotic as treatment for the ulcer? If so, • What is the name of the antibiotic? • How long do you have to take it? • Are you having any ill effects from the antibiotic?

(continued)

(continued)

Health Problem	Question
	Are you taking any other medicine for the ulcers? ● Do you have to get a vitamin injection every month because of the ulcers?
	Have you been told to avoid certain things because of the ulcer, such as: ● Aspirin? ● Other over-the-counter pain medicine? ● Alcohol? ● Smoking?
	Have you ever been hospitalized because the ulcers were bleeding? ● If so, when was the last time this happened?
	For what reasons have you been directed by your doctor or health care provider to seek additional medical care because of the ulcers?
Small bowel obstruction	When were you told you had an obstruction in your small intestine?
	What were you told was the reason the obstruction occurred?
	What symptoms did you have/ are you having now because of the obstruction such as: ● Abdominal pain? ● Bloating? ● Constipation?
	What treatment have you been prescribed for the obstruction?

(continued)

(continued)

Health Problem	Question
	Are you scheduled for/planning to have surgery for the obstruction? If so, • When is this going to be done/ when was it done?
	For what reasons have you been directed by your doctor or health care provider to seek additional medical care because of the ulcers?
Irritable bowel syndrome	When were you told you have irritable bowel syndrome?
	What are your symptoms? Such as: • Abdominal pain? • Periods of diarrhea and then periods of constipation? • Hard lumpy stool? • Bloating? • Excessive flatus/gas?
	What medicine have you been taking for the irritable bowel syndrome? • Has the medication improved the symptoms?
	What other changes have you made because of the irritable bowel syndrome such as: • Increasing the amount of fiber that you eat? • Avoiding milk or dairy products? • Avoiding foods such as beans, cabbage, apples, and nuts? • Avoiding all caffeine and caffein-ated drinks?
	For what reasons have you been directed by your doctor or health care provider to seek additional medical care because of the irritable bowel syndrome?

(continued)

(continued)

Health Problem	Question
Ulcerative colitis	When were you told that you have this disorder?
	What are your symptoms? Such as • Diarrhea (four to six stools a day)? • Fever? • Rectal bleeding? • Mucus in the stool?
	What medicine are you taking for the ulcerative colitis? • Is the medication helping?
	What other things have you changed because of the ulcerative colitis, such as: • Eliminating dairy products (milk, cheese, yogurt)? • Increasing roughage by eating fruit and vegetables?
	Has your doctor or health care professional said anything about needing surgery for the problem?
	For what reasons have you been directed by your doctor or health care provider to seek additional medical care because of the ulcerative colitis?
Crohn's disease	When were you told that you have this disease?
	What symptoms of the disease are you having right now? • Constant diarrhea? • Abdominal pain? • Weight loss? • Loss of appetite? • Nausea? • Vomiting?
	What medicine are you taking for the disease? Is it helping?

(continued)

(continued)

Health Problem	Question
	What other things have you changed because of the disease? Such as: • Avoiding all foods with roughage or fiber? • Drinking liquid supplements?
	Have you ever had surgery because of the disease? If so, when was this done? • Was some of your bowel removed? • Do you have an ostomy (ileostomy, colostomy)? • Where is the ostomy located? • What is the consistency of the stool that comes out of the ostomy? • Are you having any problems with the skin around the ostomy? • Are you able to change the ostomy appliance yourself?
	For what reasons have you been directed by your doctor or health care provider to seek additional medical care because of the Crohn's disease?
Diverticulitis/Diverticulosis	When were you told that you have diverticulitis/diverticulosis?
	What were your symptoms? • Pain after eating foods with seeds such as popcorn, nuts, strawberries?
	What treatment were you prescribed for the health problem? • Increase roughage? • Avoid roughage?
	What medicine are you taking for the health problem?
	Have you ever been in the hospital for the health problem?

(continued)

(continued)

Health Problem	Question
	For what reasons have you been directed by your doctor or health care provider to seek additional medical care because of the diverticulitis/diverticulosis?
Appendicitis	When were you told that you had appendicitis?
	What were your symptoms? ⦁ Abdominal pain (that got worse with walking or coughing)?
	What treatment did you have for the appendicitis?
	Did you have surgery to remove the appendix? If so, when was this done?
	Did you have any fevers or an infection after the appendix was removed?
	For what reasons have you been directed by your doctor or health care provider to seek additional medical care because of the appendix problem? (Keep in mind that the pain of appendicitis can be severe. If the pain suddenly stops or disappears, the appendix could have ruptured. This is an emergency situation requiring surgery to prevent peritonitis.)
Hemorrhoids	When were you told that you have hemorrhoids?
	When did you first notice a problem? Was it: ⦁ After having a baby? ⦁ Associated with constipation? ⦁ After a weight gain? ⦁ Sitting too long at work? ⦁ Eating a low-fiber diet?

(continued)

(continued)

Health Problem	Question
	What symptoms do you have because of the hemorrhoids?
	What medicine do you use for the hemorrhoids? • Does the medicine help?
	Have you been told that you need surgery for the hemorrhoids? If so, when was it/will it be done?
	Have you had to make any other changes because of the hemorrhoids?
	For what reasons have you been directed by your doctor or health care provider to seek additional medical care because of the hemorrhoids?
Liver cirrhosis	When were you told that you have liver cirrhosis?
	What were you told was the reason that the condition developed?
	What symptoms are you experiencing right now? Such as: • Abdominal swelling? • Bleeding (in the stool or in vomit)? • Bruising? • Jaundice? • Loss of appetite? • Diarrhea?
	Have you been in the hospital for the cirrhosis? Was it because of bleeding from your stomach or esophagus?
	What medicine are you taking for the cirrhosis, such as: • Water pill (diuretic)? • Antibiotics? • Lactulose? • Vitamin supplements? • Antacids?

(continued)

(continued)

Health Problem	Question
	What other treatment have you been prescribed for the cirrhosis such as: ◦ Low-salt diet? ◦ Avoiding all alcohol?
	For what reasons have you been directed by your doctor or health care provider to seek additional medical care because of the cirrhosis?
Hepatitis	When were you told that you have/ had hepatitis?
	What type of hepatitis were you told that you had/have? A, B, or C?
	What were you told was the reason you developed hepatitis? ◦ Ingesting food that was infected with fecal material? ◦ Exposure to blood?
	What symptoms are you currently experiencing? ◦ Jaundice? ◦ Fatigue? ◦ Weakness? ◦ Loss of appetite? ◦ Abdominal pain?
	What medicine are you taking for the hepatitis?
	Were you given vaccinations to prevent any future episodes of hepatitis?
	Were you prescribed any other treatment for the hepatitis?
	For what reasons have you been directed by your doctor or health care provider to seek additional medical care because of the hepatitis?

(continued)

(continued)

Health Problem	Question
Cholelithiasis/Cholecystitis	When were you told that you have a problem with your gallbladder?
	What were you told was/is the problem? • Infection? • Inflammation? • Stones in the gallbladder? • Rapid weight loss? • Use of medications?
	What symptoms are you having right now because of your gallbladder? • Right shoulder pain? • Nausea? • Vomiting? • Abdominal pain? • Stool appears clay colored?
	What medicine have you been taking for the gallbladder problem? Is it helping with the pain?
	What other things are you doing to help with the gall bladder problem: • Avoiding high-fat foods?
	Are you scheduled for/planning to have surgery to remove your gallbladder? • When was it/when is it going to be done?
	For what reasons have you been directed by your doctor or health care provider to seek additional medical care because of your gallbladder?
Pancreatitis	When were you told that you have a problem with your pancreas?
	What were you told was the reason that you have a problem with your pancreas?

(continued)

(*continued*)

Health Problem	Question
	What symptoms are you having right now because of your pancreas? ◉ Abdominal pain that radiates to your back? ◉ Pain after eating a high-fat meal or drinking alcohol? ◉ Nausea? ◉ Vomiting? ◉ Bloating?
	What medicine are you taking for your pancreas? ◉ Pain medication? ◉ Enzyme replacements? Is it helping with the symptoms?
	What else have you been directed to do to help with your pancreas problem? ◉ Low-fat diet? ◉ Avoiding all alcohol?
	For what reasons have you been directed by your doctor or health care provider to seek additional medical care because of your pancreas?
Eating disorder: anorexia nervosa/ bulimia nervosa	The patient/client may not refer to this disorder with the appropriate name. It may be referred to as not eating or avoiding food. For bulimia, it might be referred to as binge eating or vomiting after eating.
	When did you realize that you have a problem with eating food?
	What happens when you eat food? ◉ How do you feel when you eat food? (Keep in mind that the assessment does not go in depth into the psychology of anorexia nervosa.)

(*continued*)

(*continued*)

Health Problem	Question
	Do you ever make yourself throw up after eating? • How does that make you feel? • How often do you do this? • Are you having any problems because of throwing up such as: ▪ Problems with your teeth? ▪ Sore throat?
	Have you ever been hospitalized because you were not eating/throwing up too much?
	Have you ever had to have food replacements given to you through your veins or through a tube that goes into the stomach?
	How are you feeling right now? When was the last time that you ate something/felt the need to throw up?
	For what reasons have you been directed by your doctor or health care provider to seek additional medical care because of your eating problem?

SUGGESTIONS FOR GASTROINTESTINAL DISORDERS

● Find out the term or words the client uses to describe the problem. Some clients may not want to say "diarrhea" or "constipation." Alternative terms might be "loose bowels" or having problems with "doing a job."

● Ask first how the client is currently feeling with the health problem. Usual symptoms can be assessed afterward.

● Determine if the client is prescribed any specific medication or treatment for the health problem. Ask if the client has been adhering to what has been prescribed and if the treatment or medication has helped. If the client is not adhering to the prescribed treatment or medication, find out why. Brainstorm ways with the client to help improve adherence if possible.

- Reinforce prescribed treatment or therapy. Do not suggest alternative treatment approaches.
- Once the acute/chronic gastrointestinal problem has been assessed, find out if the client is having any other problems.
- Listen for the client's responses to your questions. They may not want to talk directly about the health problem but mention it with other health issues. For example, a patient/client may say that they can't tolerate milk because it makes the stomach hurt and causes diarrhea.
- It is unlikely that a client with stomach/colon cancer will be enrolled in a disease management program. If you learn that a client has this disease process, any of the questions suggested for the other gastrointestinal health problems would be appropriate to use for an assessment.
- Be sure to give the client sufficient time to discuss the problem, medications, treatments, or any other therapy to prevent exacerbation of the health problem.

PRACTICE EXERCISES

Read the following client situations and determine:

- Which questions to ask
- What the client might be experiencing
- Whether the situation requires the client to contact the doctor or health care provider

1. A middle-aged adult client experiences diarrhea for 3 or 4 days and then has a period of constipation for about a week. Then the cycle repeats.
2. A patient with a history of stomach ulcers has new mouth sores and asks if mouthwash could be used to heal them.
3. A client who started a new job a few months ago is experiencing abdominal pain, cramping, and excessive flatus that is relieved after having a bowel movement. If unable to have a bowel movement, the client uses a rapid-acting laxative.
4. A client with GERD has been avoiding eating for several days and experiences severe abdominal pain after eating pizza and drinking beer.

5. A client with a history of hepatitis asks why the skin feels so itchy.
6. A client with a history of appendicitis says that the pain was really severe a short while ago but suddenly stopped.
7. During an assessment, a patient with liver cirrhosis sounds confused and mentions the inability to have bowel movements for several days.

CASE STUDY

Bob is a telephonic nurse for an organization that provides disease management services. The next client to contact is a 35-year-old female with a long-standing history of Crohn's disease.

- What is the first question that should be asked?
- What response should cause you to focus on the quality of the client's bowel movements?

The client says that for the last several days the amount of diarrhea has been increasing and is having a new problem with leg cramps. She asks if she should rub her legs or put on support hose to help this.

- What might be occurring with this client?
- What advice should be given to this client right now?

Bob notes that the client has not responded to messages left for two subsequent care calls. Later in the day, the client calls into the office and reports having just been discharged from the hospital for bowel surgery.

- What questions would be the most important to ask first?
- What situations would cause you to think that the client was having a complication after the surgery.

During the conversation the client asks when the bowel movement in the "bag" is going to become firm because she is "tired" of always having diarrhea. Bob notes that claims have been paid for a partial colectomy with the placement of a transverse colostomy.

How would you respond to this client's question about the type of bowel movement?

What discharge information would be essential for you to have?

A week later, Bob learns that the client is having skin ulceration and soreness at the site of the ostomy appliance. The client wants to leave the appliance off and just use gauze pads to collect the stool.

How should this client's plan be addressed?

What should you suggest that the client do at this time?

KEY POINTS

Gastrointestinal disorders can occur anywhere along the alimentary tract, beginning with the mouth and ending with the rectum and anus.

Many people find talking about this body system and the associated diseases as highly personal and may hesitate to answer direct questions.

Patients/clients with gastrointestinal disorders often do not have difficulty with talking on the telephone but may want to change the subject.

Remember to reinforce the prescribed treatment and medications for the health problem. Do not recommend any complementary or alternative therapies. If the patient/client asks about the use of herbs or vitamins to treat the disorder, refer him or her to the health care professional.

BIBLIOGRAPHY

D'Amico, D., & Barbarito, C. (2012). *Health and physical assessment in nursing* (2nd ed.). Upper Saddle River, NJ: Pearson.

Lemone, P. (2015). *Medical-surgical nursing* (6th ed.). Upper Saddle River, NJ: Pearson.

Pearson Education (2015). *Nursing: A concept-based approach to learning* (2nd ed., Vol. 2). Upper Saddle River, NJ: Author.

CHAPTER 16

Disorders of the Musculoskeletal System

Upon completion of this chapter, the nurse will:

1. Summarize the different disorders of the musculoskeletal system
2. Examine approaches to assess different disorders of the musculoskeletal system
3. Determine approaches that can be used for more than one musculoskeletal disorder

MUSCULOSKELETAL DISORDERS

Disorders of the musculoskeletal system can range from minor ailments to more severe chronic conditions. The disorders identified are the most common ones appropriate for telephonic care and include:

- Sprain
- Repetitive use injury
- Fracture
- Amputation
- Osteoporosis
- Gout
- Osteoarthritis
- Post-polio syndrome
- Rheumatoid arthritis
- Ankylosing spondylitis
- Spinal stenosis
- Osteomyelitis

- Back pain
- Fibromyalgia
- Spinal deformity
- Foot disorders

ASSESSING DISORDERS OF THE MUSCULOSKELETAL SYSTEM

Remember that the client is already diagnosed with a musculoskeletal problem. When providing telephonic care, you are assessing the client's current condition, symptoms, and if anything has changed or needs to be referred to the doctor/health care professional.

Health Problem	Question
Sprain	When were you told that you had a sprain?
	Where is the sprain located?
	When did the sprain occur?
	What were you told to do to treat the sprain? (RICE) ● Rest? ● Ice? ● Compression? ● Elevation?
	Are you able to walk with the sprain?
	What are you doing to treat the pain?
	For what reasons have you been directed by your doctor or health care provider to seek additional medical care because of the sprain?
Repetitive use injury	When were you told that you have a repetitive use injury?
	Where is it located?
	What are your symptoms? ● Pain? ● Numbness? ● Tingling?
	How long have you had this injury?

(continued)

(continued)

Health Problem	Question
	What are you doing for the injury? ◦ Avoiding certain activity? ◦ Using a splint? ◦ Taking over-the-counter analgesics?
	Have you been told that you might need surgery? ◦ If so, when is this going to occur?
	For what reasons have you been directed by your doctor or health care provider to seek additional medical care because of the injury?
Dislocation	What joint was dislocated?
	When did it happen?
	How did it happen?
	Was the joint "put back into the socket"? (closed reduction)
	What were you told to do to treat it? ◦ Pain medication? ◦ Splinting? ◦ Mild range of motion exercises?
	For what reasons have you been directed by your doctor/health care provider to seek additional medical care because of the injury?
Fracture	What bone was broken (fractured)?
	When did it happen?
	How did it happen?
	What has been done to treat it? ◦ Casting? ◦ Surgery? ◦ Splinting?
	If casted, what have you been directed to do to care for the cast such as: ◦ Report if the cast feels tight? ◦ Make sure the cast does not get wet? ◦ Place nothing down the cast to scratch itchy skin?

(continued)

Health Problem	Question
	How long do you need to wear the cast?
	Have you been told that you will need physical therapy after the cast is removed?
	(If a lower extremity is casted) What are you using to help you walk? ● Crutches? ● Cane? ● Walker?
	When do you go back to have the broken bone checked?
	For what reasons have you been directed by your doctor or health care provider to seek additional medical care because of the broken bone?
Amputation	When did you have your (leg/arm) amputated?
	Can you tell me why it needed to be amputated?
	How long ago was that done?
	Has your stump healed?
	Have you been fitted for a prosthesis? ● Are you wearing it?
	(If below knee amputation) Are you doing any exercises to make sure your knee can be bent and straightened?
	(If above knee amputation) Were you directed to lie on your stomach on the bed for short periods of time every day to make sure your hip joints do not get tight?
	Are you having any pain in your leg/arm with the amputation? (Might experience phantom limb pain.) If so, ● What are you doing to help with the pain? ● Is it helping? Does it control the pain?
	When are you supposed to go back and see the surgeon for the amputation?
	For what reasons have you been directed by your doctor or health care provider to seek additional medical care because of the amputation?

(continued)

(*continued*)

Health Problem	Question
Osteoporosis	Who told you that you have osteoporosis?
	How was it diagnosed?
	How long ago were you told?
	What medicine are you taking for the osteoporosis? Are you taking the medicine as prescribed such as: ◦ Taking it in the morning with a full glass of water on an empty stomach? ◦ Sitting upright for 30 minutes after taking the medication?
	Are you supposed to take calcium and vitamin D supplements also?
	Have you been directed to do anything to help with the osteoporosis such as: ◦ Engaging in weight-bearing exercise (walking)? ◦ Smoking cessation? ◦ Avoiding alcohol intake?
	Have you had any broken bones because of the osteoporosis? If so, ◦ Which one(s): ▪ Hip? ▪ Femur? ▪ Vertebrae?
	When are you supposed to see your doctor again for the osteoporosis?
	For what reasons have you been directed by your doctor/health care provider to seek additional medical care because of the osteoporosis?
Gout	When were you told that you have gout?
	Where is the gout located? ◦ Foot? ◦ Toe? ◦ Knee?
	What are/were your symptoms: ◦ Pain? ◦ Swelling?

(*continued*)

(continued)

Health Problem	Question
	What medicine are you taking for the gout? ● Are you taking it as directed?
	What else are you doing to treat the gout? ● Change in diet? (avoiding foods high in purines) ● Avoiding alcohol?
	When are you supposed to see your doctor again for the gout?
	For what reasons have you been directed by your doctor or health care provider to seek additional medical care because of the gout?
Back pain	When did you start to have back pain?
	How long has it been going on?
	Were you doing anything in particular when it started? Such as: ● Lifting heavy item? ● Twisting the torso?
	What have you been doing to treat the back pain, such as: ● Rest? ● Ice/heat? ● Mild exercise? ● Over-the-counter pain medicine?
	Were you told the reason for the back pain, such as: ● Slipped/herniated disk?
	Are you having any problems, such as: ● Limb weakness? ● Numbness? ● Tingling? ● Change in bowel or bladder function?
	Were you told that you need/did you have surgery for the back pain? If so, ● When is this going to be done/when did you have it done?
	When are you supposed to see your doctor again for the back pain?

(continued)

(continued)

Health Problem	Question
	For what reasons have you been directed by your doctor or health care provider to seek additional medical care because of the back pain?
Spinal deformity	What kind of spinal problem do you have? Such as: ● Scoliosis? ● Kyphosis? ● Lordosis?
	What have you been directed to do for the spinal deformity? ● Physical therapy? ● Wear a back brace? ● Avoid twisting the torso (avoid golfing)? ● Avoid activities that could cause falls such as climbing a ladder, riding a horse?
	Are you experiencing any other problems because of the spinal deformity, such as: ● Difficulty breathing? ● Issues with bowel function?
	How often do you see your doctor because of the spinal deformity? ● When is your next appointment?
	For what reasons have you been directed by your doctor/health care provider to seek additional medical care because of the spinal deformity?
Ankylosing spondylitis/ spinal stenosis	When were you told that you have ankylosing spondylitis/spinal stenosis?
	What tests did you have done to diagnose the disorder? ● MRI? ● Myelogram? ● CT Scan?
	What symptoms are you having now?

(continued)

(*continued*)

Health Problem	Question
	What have you been told to do to help with the problem? • Exercises/physical therapy? • Swimming? • Weight reduction? • Smoking cessation? • Apply ice/heat?
	What medicine are you using to treat the pain? • Over-the-counter pain medicine? • Prescribed pain medicine?
	Have you been told to avoid doing anything because of the problem, such as: • Avoid heavy lifting? • Avoid twisting the torso?
	Have you been told that you might need surgery for the problem? If so, • When is this going to be done/when was it done?
	When are you going to see your doctor again for the problem?
	For what reasons have you been directed by your doctor/health care provider to seek additional medical care because of the problem?
Osteoarthritis/ rheumatoid arthritis	When were you told you have arthritis? What type of arthritis do you have?
	How long have you had this problem?
	What areas on your body are affected, such as: • Hips? • Knees? • Spine? • Hands?

	What symptoms do you have?
	• Osteoarthritis:
	  ▪ Morning stiffness?
	  ▪ Joint pain?
	• Rheumatoid arthritis:
	  ▪ Joint pain?
	  ▪ Joint swelling?
	  ▪ Fever?

(*continued*)

(continued)

Health Problem	Question

	What do you do to help with the symptoms?
	• Osteoarthritis:
	  ▪ Exercise?
	  ▪ Weight reduction?
	  ▪ Heat?
	• Rheumatoid arthritis:
	  ▪ Rest?
	  ▪ Ice?

	What medicine do you take for the arthritis? • Nonsteroidal anti-inflammatory drugs (NSAIDs)? • Prescribed pain killers?
	Have you been told that you might need to have a joint replaced because of the arthritis? If so, • Which joint? • When is this going to be done? • Have you had other joints replaced because of the arthritis?
	When are you supposed to see your doctor again for the arthritis?
	For what reasons have you been directed by your doctor or health care provider to seek additional medical care because of the arthritis?
Fibromyalgia	When were you told that you have fibromyalgia?
	What body areas are the most affected?
	What are your symptoms, such as: • Muscle pain? • Problems with sleeping?
	How long have you been having these symptoms?
	What have you been doing to help with the problem, such as: • Exercise? • Rest periods? • Weight reduction? • Stress reduction? • Dietary changes? • Vitamin supplements?

(continued)

(*continued*)

Health Problem	Question
	What medicine, if any, have you been prescribed for the problem?
	What over-the-counter preparations do you take for the problem?
	When are you supposed to see your doctor again for the problem?
	For what reasons have you been directed by your doctor/health care provider to seek additional medical care because of the fibromyalgia?
Osteomyelitis	When were you told that you have a bone infection?
	What caused the infection, such as: ● After surgery? ● Injury? ● Other illness?
	What has been done to treat the infection, such as: ● Surgery? ● Wound care? ● Pain medication? ● Antibiotics?
	Who helps you do your wound dressing?
	Do you have visiting nurses to help with the dressing?
	How long were you told that you need to take antibiotics for the infection?
	When are you supposed to see your doctor again for the infection?
	For what reasons have you been directed by your doctor or health care provider to seek additional medical care because of the infection?
Post-polio syndrome	(The polio vaccination was provided to the general public in the 1960s. At that time, a derivative of the live poliovirus was administered, and some individuals reacted to the virus causing a mild form of polio. Individuals who were diagnosed with polio were treated and for years had no problems. Over time as some of these individuals aged, symptoms of the disorder resurfaced leading to the health problem post-polio syndrome. Other people who experienced polio in their youth can also develop this syndrome.)

(*continued*)

(continued)

Health Problem	Question
	When did you have polio?
	When did you notice that you were having symptoms of the problem again?
	What are you experiencing? ● Muscle weakness/limb weakness? ● Pain? ● Numbness? ● Tingling?
	What have you been doing for the symptoms? ● Exercise? ● Rest? ● Dietary changes? ● Symptom treatment with medicine?
	How are you feeling right now?
	What has your doctor told you about the problem?
	When do you see your doctor again for the problem?
	For what reasons have you been directed by your doctor/health care provider to seek additional medical care because of the problem?
Foot disorders	What type of foot problem do you have? ● Hammertoe? ● Bunion? ● Neuroma? ● Heel pain?
	How long have you had this problem?
	What have you been doing to treat the problem? ● Orthotics? ● Surgery? ● Wearing different shoes?
	Have you been told that you need surgery to correct the foot problem? ● Are you going to have the surgery/did you have the surgery?
	When do you see your doctor again for the foot problem?
	For what reasons have you been directed by your doctor or health care provider to seek additional medical care because of the foot problem?

SUGGESTIONS FOR MUSCULOSKELETAL DISORDERS

- Remember that not all patients will know the name of their disorder. Older patients/clients may refer to all aches and pains as arthritis.
- Begin care calls with asking how the patient is feeling right now. Before engaging in a lengthy conversation, ask if they are comfortable sitting. Prolonged sitting can aggravate arthritic hips and knees.
- Take the time to instruct or reinforce home safety approaches. Find out if the patient has grab bars in the bathroom near the shower and commode. Remind to remove throw rugs and keep clutter off of the floors and stairways. Reinforce the need to always wear footwear both inside and outside of the home.
- Should a patient use an assistive device to walk, ask if the device has been properly fitted and that they are using it appropriately.
- The frequency of calls after orthopedic surgery might be more frequently scheduled. These calls can continue even if the patient is receiving home care.
- Always find out first what the health care provider has prescribed as treatment for the disorder. Remember to never suggest a treatment, medication, or supplement. Many patients with musculoskeletal disorders will be taking calcium and vitamin D supplements. Your role is to encourage the patient to take the supplements as prescribed even though the patient will not "see" the supplement working. They are used to prevent future bone conditions.
- Some patients may be isolated because of their musculoskeletal problem and look forward to the telephone calls. Keep a conversational approach and encourage the patient to express feelings.
- It is unlikely that a patient with primary or metastatic bone cancer will be enrolled in a disease management program.

PRACTICE EXERCISES

Read the following client situations and determine:

- Which questions to ask
- What the client might be experiencing
- Whether the situation requires the client to contact the doctor or health care provider

1. A client recovering from knee replacement surgery asks if it is normal for her leg to feel numb.
2. During an assessment, a client with osteoarthritis asks what it means when his bowel movements appear black in color.
3. A client with a cast on the lower right leg reports using a coat hanger to scratch the skin under the cast because it has become so itchy in the summer heat.
4. An older patient with rheumatoid arthritis wants to know if it would be all right to take a bus trip with the senior citizen's group.
5. While conducting an assessment, a client in a wellness program asks what it means when the body aches all of the time.
6. A client in a wellness program asks what can be done to reduce the numbness and tingling in her right hand while working on the computer at work.
7. A client returning home after hip replacement surgery becomes short of breath during a care call.
8. An older client being treated for gout states a plan to meet up with friends at the local bar to watch the football game later in the evening.
9. An older client recovering from a spinal fracture from osteoporosis lights a cigarette during a care call.
10. A client with an amputation above the left knee says that the limb prosthesis is uncomfortable because of a sore on the stump.

CASE STUDY

A client enrolled in the diabetes disease management program has not been able to be reached for several weeks. Ginny, the telephonic nurse, contacts the health insurance company to learn that the client is currently in rehabilitation after an amputation below the right knee. The estimated day of discharge is in a week.

- What information should be prepared to help this client recover successfully at home?
- What guidance should be provided to help prevent additional amputations in the future?

The client returns home and takes the next call from Ginny. He explains that he had a foot sore for several months that was not healing and the doctors decided that an amputation was needed. The client is experiencing "severe" pain and wants to rub the foot on the amputated limb.

- How should you explain this type of pain to the client?
- What suggestions could be made to help the client reduce the pain?

In a few weeks, the client calls in and says that the limb pain has gotten better, but he asks what should be done because the stump is swollen and the prosthesis is feeling tight. He has tried wrapping the stump with an elastic bandage, but it made the stump ache.

- What additional information do you need?
- What direction should you provide at this time?

Two weeks later, Ginny sees that the client had a claim paid for an outpatient procedure to drain a hematoma from the stump. During the care call, the client says that there was bleeding in the stump, which caused it to swell and asks when he can use the prosthesis again.

- What additional information should you obtain from the client now?
- How should you answer the question about the use of the prosthesis?

KEY POINTS

- People of all ages can have musculoskeletal disorders. These disorders do not just affect older individuals.
- Approach the assessment of this body system methodically. Skip any areas that are not applicable based on client responses.
- If asked "what to do" about any disorder, find out what the health care provider has prescribed for treatment. Reinforcing the health care provider's treatment plan is essential. Never suggest a complementary or alternative therapy approach.
- Remember to assess the home environment for potential safety issues, particularly if a client is not receiving home care services. Home care nurses will conduct home safety assessments; however, not all clients recovering or experiencing musculoskeletal disorders will have this service.

- Clients with chronic ailments such as arthritis may become depressed because of the ongoing pain and stiffness. Gently encourage these clients to follow their treatment plan and help them to stay positive.
- Be aware that bed rest or inactivity is not recommended as treatment for low back pain. These clients may resist performing exercises. Remind that inactivity can slow the recovery and make movement more difficult.
- Always find out what the client has been directed to do regarding activity before discussing exercises.
- For any clients who use assistive devices, find out if the device was fitted by physical therapy. People may just "buy a cane" at the local pharmacy and it is not of the correct height. Using a device that has not been fitted could cause additional problems.

BIBLIOGRAPHY

D'Amico, D., & Barbarito, C., (2012). *Health and physical assessment in nursing* (2nd ed.). Upper Saddle River, NJ: Pearson.

Lemone, P. (2015). *Medical-surgical nursing* (6th ed.). Upper Saddle River, NJ: Pearson.

Pearson Education. (2015). *Nursing: A concept-based approach to learning* (2nd ed., Vol. 2). Upper Saddle River, NJ: Author.

CHAPTER 17

Disorders of the Neurologic and Sensory Systems

LEARNING OUTCOMES

Upon completion of this chapter, the nurse will:

1. Summarize the different disorders of the neurologic and sensory systems
2. Examine approaches to assess different disorders of the neurologic and sensory systems
3. Determine approaches that can be used for more than one neurologic or sensory disorder

NEUROLOGIC AND SENSORY SYSTEM DISORDERS

Disorders of the neurologic and sensory systems can range from a sudden onset of acute symptoms indicating a severe problem to chronic diseases. The ones that would be the most appropriate for telephonic care include:

- Seizure disorders
- Stroke
- Concussion
- Headaches
  - Tension
  - Cluster
  - Migraine
- Spinal cord injury
- Herniated disk
- Multiple sclerosis
- Parkinson's disease

- Myasthenia gravis
- Trigeminal neuralgia
- Bell's palsy
- Cataracts
- Glaucoma
- Macular degeneration
- Detached retina
- Deafness/hearing loss

ASSESSING DISORDERS OF THE NEUROLOGIC AND SENSORY SYSTEMS

Remember that the client most likely is already diagnosed with a neurologic or sensory system problem. The focus of the call should be on assessing the client's current status and if there have been any recent changes.

Health Problem	Changes
Seizure disorder	When were you told that you have a seizure disorder?
	What type of seizures do you have? • Tonic-clonic (grand mal)? • Partial? • Absence?
	How often do you have a seizure? • When was the last one? • Does your family know what to do if/when you have a seizure?
	What medicine do you take for the seizures? • How often do you take it? • Do you have to have blood work done because of your medicine? • When was the blood work last done?
	When are you supposed to see your doctor or health care provider again for the seizures?
	For what reasons have you been directed by your doctor or health care provider to seek additional medical care because of the seizures?

(continued)

(*continued*)

Health Problem	Changes
Stroke	When did you have the stroke?
	What side of the body did the stroke affect?
	What weakness are you still experiencing?
	What other problems are you having because of the stroke, such as: ● Problems eating and swallowing? ● Controlling bowels/bladder? ● Walking/balance?
	What do you use, if anything, for safety when walking?
	What medicine have you been taking since the stroke? ● How often do you take it? ● Do you need to have blood work done because of the medicine?
	When are you supposed to see your doctor or health care provider again for the stroke?
	For what reasons have you been directed by your doctor or health care provider to seek additional medical care because of the stroke?
Concussion	When did you have the head injury?
	What were you doing when you had the injury? ● Sports activity? ● Motor vehicle accident? ● Fall?
	What symptoms are you experiencing because of the injury?
	Are you taking any medicine because of the injury? If so, ● What is the name of the medicine? ● How often do you take it?
	Are you having any kind of therapy because of the injury, such as ● Physical therapy? ● Occupational therapy?

(*continued*)

(continued)

Health Problem	Changes
	When are you supposed to see your doctor or health care provider again for the injury?
	For what reasons have you been directed by your doctor or health care provider to seek additional medical care because of the injury?
Headaches	What type of headaches do you have? ○ Tension? ○ Migraine? ○ Cluster?
	How often do they occur?
	What symptoms do you have with the headaches, such as: ○ Pain in the neck/shoulders (tension)? ○ Eye pain and tearing (cluster)? ○ Photophobia, nausea, vomiting (migraine)?
	What medicine are you taking for the headaches? ○ How often do you take the medicine? ○ Is the medicine effective?
	Is there anything that you were told to do to help prevent the headaches, such as: ○ Increasing activity/exercise (tension)? ○ Avoid alcohol, chocolate, caffeine (migraine)? ○ Smoking cessation? Has avoiding these things helped?
	When are you supposed to see your doctor or health care provider again for the headaches?
	For what reasons have you been directed by your doctor or health care provider to seek additional medical care because of the headaches?
Spinal cord injury/nerve compression	When did you have the injury?
	What symptoms are you having now/still experiencing, such as: ○ Numbness? ○ Tingling? ○ Paralysis?

(continued)

(continued)

Health Problem	Changes
	Do you have any other problems that were caused by the injury, such as: • Problems with your bowels or bladder? • Muscle cramping?
	Were you prescribed any medicine to help with the symptoms of the injury? If so, • What is the name of the medicine? • How often do you take it? • Has it been effective to control the symptoms?
	When are you supposed to see your doctor or health care provider again for the injury/nerve compression?
	For what reasons have you been directed by your doctor or health care provider to seek additional medical care because of the injury/nerve compression?
Herniated disk/ back surgery	When did you have the herniated disk/back surgery?
	What symptoms are you having right now, such as: • Pain? • Spasms? • Muscle weakness?
	What medicine are you taking for the problem? • Is the medicine effective?
	What else have you been prescribed for the problem, such as: • Physical therapy? • Water therapy? • Transcutaneous electrical nerve stimulation (TENS) unit? • Back brace? • Smoking cessation? • Weight reduction/management?
	When are you supposed to see your doctor or health care provider again for the disk injury/back surgery?
	For what reasons have you been directed by your doctor or health care provider to seek additional medical care because of the disk injury/back surgery?

(continued)

(continued)

Health Problem	Changes
Multiple sclerosis	When were you told you have multiple sclerosis?
	What symptoms do you have right now, such as: ● Vision changes? ● Problems walking or using your hands? ● Problems with bowel/bladder control? ● Overall weakness?
	What do you use for help with self-care and mobility, such as: ● Splints? ● Walker? ● Wheelchair?
	What else were you told to do to help with the symptoms, such as: ● Frequent rest periods? ● Avoid extremes in temperature? ● Weight management?
	What medicine do you take for the symptoms? ● Is the medicine effective?
	When are you supposed to see your doctor or health care provider again for the health problem?
	For what reasons have you been directed by your doctor or health care provider to seek additional medical care because of the health problem?
Parkinson's disease	When were you told that you have this disorder?
	What symptoms are you having now, such as: ● Hand tremor? ● Stiffness of the arms and legs? ● Problems with walking?
	Are you having any problems with: ● Eating? ● Swallowing? ● Breathing? ● Sweating? ● Having bowel movements?

(continued)

(*continued*)

Health Problem	Changes
	What medicine do you take for the health problem? ◦ How often do you take it? ◦ Has it helped with your health problem?
	When are you supposed to see your doctor or health care provider again for the health problem?
	For what reasons have you been directed by your doctor or health care provider to seek additional medical care because of the health problem?
Myasthenia gravis	When were you told that you have myasthenia gravis?
	What symptoms are you having right now, such as: ◦ Difficulty talking? ◦ Problems with swallowing? ◦ Weak voice? ◦ Difficulty writing or doing other activities with the hands?
	Were you told to do anything else to help with the symptoms, such as: ◦ Avoiding extreme temperatures? ◦ Getting enough rest?

	What medicine are you taking for the health problem?
	◦ How often do you take it?
	◦ Do you keep a supply of extra doses in your (purse, pocket)?
	◦ What happens if you take too much of the medicine?
	  ▪ What are you supposed to do if that happens?
	◦ What happens if you miss a dose or several doses of the medicine?
	  ▪ What are you supposed to do if that happens?

	When are you supposed to see your doctor or health care provider again for the health problem?
	For what reasons have you been directed by your doctor or health care provider to seek additional medical care because of the health problem?

(*continued*)

(*continued*)

Health Problem	Changes
Trigeminal neuralgia/tic douloureux	When were you told you have this problem?
	What symptoms are you having right now, such as: • Eye tearing? • Eye pain? • Face/jaw pain?
	What treatment have you had for the problem, such as: • Surgery? • Medication?
	If you are taking medication, how effective has it been?
	When are you supposed to see your doctor or health care provider again for the health problem?
	For what reasons have you been directed by your doctor or health care provider to seek additional medical care because of the health problem?
Bell's palsy/facial paralysis	When were you told that you have facial paralysis/Bell's palsy?
	What symptoms are you having right now, such as: • Continued facial weakness? • Problems closing the eye on the side of the face with the weakness?
	What have you been told to do for the symptoms, such as: • Massage the face muscles? • Apply warm compresses to the face? • Use artificial tears in the eyes? • Eat a soft diet? • Perform facial exercises?
	When are you supposed to see your doctor or health care provider again for the paralysis?
	For what reasons have you been directed by your doctor or health care provider to seek additional medical care because of the paralysis?

(*continued*)

(*continued*)

Health Problem	Changes
Cataracts	Where were you told that you have a cataract?
	What symptoms are you experiencing right now, such as: ● Cloudy vision? ● Glare? ● Problems seeing the color blue?
	When are you having surgery to remove the cataract?
	If postoperative: When did you have the surgery to remove the cataract? ● What eye drops are you taking after the surgery? ● Did you have a lens implanted with the surgery? ● When are you supposed to see the doctor again after the surgery?
	Were you told that you have a cataract developing in your other eye?
	Were you told when you might need surgery on the cataract in the other eye?
	For what reasons have you been directed by your doctor or health care provider to seek additional medical care because of the cataract?
Glaucoma	When were you told that you have glaucoma?
	What symptoms are you having right now, such as: ● Reduced vision? ● Eye pain?
	What medicine are you taking for the glaucoma?
	Are you going to have/had surgery for the glaucoma? ● When is it going to be done/when was it done? ● If postoperative: What changes have you noticed in your vision since the surgery?
	When are you supposed to see your doctor or health care provider again for the glaucoma?
	For what reasons have you been directed by your doctor or health care provider to seek additional medical care because of the glaucoma?

(*continued*)

(continued)

Health Problem	Changes
Macular degeneration	When were you told that you have macular degeneration?
	What type were you told that you have: ● Wet? ● Dry?
	What symptoms do you have right now such as: ● Blurry central vision in one/both eyes? ● No changes to peripheral vision?
	Are you using any eye drops/medicine because of the problem? ● Have you noticed if the eye drops have made any difference in your vision?
	Are you planning to have/had surgery for the macular degeneration? ● When is the surgery scheduled/when did you have the surgery? ● If postoperative: have you noticed any changes in your vision since the surgery?
	When are you supposed to see your doctor or health care provider again for the macular degeneration?
	For what reasons have you been directed by your doctor or health care provider to seek additional medical care because of the macular degeneration?
Detached retina	When were you told that you had a detached retina?
	What were you doing when it happened?
	When did you have surgery to repair the retina? ● Do you know the type of surgery that you had?
	How is your vision right now?
	Are you having any other problems caused by the detached retina, such as: ● Floaters? ● Transient blindness? ● Loss of central vision?
	When are you supposed to see your doctor or health care provider again for the detached retina?

(continued)

(continued)

Health Problem	Changes
	For what reasons have you been directed by your doctor or health care provider to seek additional medical care because of the detached retina?
Deafness/hearing loss	When were you told/when did you first start to notice problems with your hearing?
	Were you told what type of hearing loss you have? ● Sensory? ● Conductive? ● Both?
	Do you have any other symptoms with the hearing loss, such as: ● Nausea/vomiting? ● Dizziness?
	What treatments have you had to help with the hearing loss, such as: ● Ear irrigation?
	What type of hearing aid do you use? ● How often do you need to change the batteries in the device(s)?
	Are you able to insert and remove the hearing aids yourself or do you need assistance?
	When are you supposed to see your doctor or health care provider again for the hearing problem?
	For what reasons have you been directed by your doctor or health care provider to seek additional medical care because of the hearing problem?

SUGGESTIONS FOR NEUROLOGIC AND SENSORY DISORDERS

● Carefully listen to the term or phrase the patient/client uses to describe or name the disorder. Use the same term when conducting the assessment.

● Remember to begin the conversation with asking how the patient is feeling right now.

● Be aware of patients who are recovering from surgery. They may not be able to conduct a lengthy care call at this time. Increase the call frequency but reduce the length of each call until the patient's endurance improves.

- Even though neurologic disorders can affect bowel and bladder functioning, some patients may not feel comfortable discussing this problem. Use general phrases such as "going too much," "going too little," or "not going at all" when discussing urine and stool output.
- Always find out the prescribed treatment for the health problem. Reinforce any prescribed treatment. If asked for an opinion regarding a complementary or alternative therapy, refer the patient back to the doctor or health care provider for discussion.
- Be sure to ask questions about home safety if the patient has a neurologic or sensory disorder that affects mobility, vision, or hearing.

PRACTICE EXERCISES

Read the following client situations and determine:

- Which questions to ask
- What the client might be experiencing
- Whether the situation requires the client to contact the doctor or health care provider

1. A client asks what it means if part of the vision of the right eye is dark.
2. A client with a history of Parkinson's disease starts to cough during the call.
3. While conducting a routine care call, an older client begins to have garbled speech and answer questions inappropriately.
4. During a postoperative care call, a client recovering from spinal fusion surgery asks if it is normal to have bladder incontinence and when the numbness in both legs might go away.
5. A client with migraine headaches asks if it would be all right to substitute a vitamin supplement for the prescribed medication.
6. A client with myasthenia gravis says that several doses of the medication were skipped because they were packed in a suitcase for travel.

7. A client with macular degeneration asks if the condition is getting better because the blurry vision has gone and has been replaced with a dark shadow area in the line of vision.
8. During a postoperative call, a client recovering from cataract surgery asks if it is normal to have blurred vision and eye pain after the surgery.
9. An older client says that the hearing aids are used sometimes because they are "hard" to get in and out of the ears. Family members need to help, and they are not always available to do so.
10. A client with glaucoma admits to not using eye drops as prescribed because "I'm not having any problems seeing and I have no pain."

CASE STUDY

Nanette, a telephonic nurse for a disease management company, is calling a client with a history of myasthenia gravis. During the call, Nanette notices that the client's voice volume is weak and asks about adhering to the prescribed medication schedule. The client says that someone is at the door and hangs up the phone.

- What should you do?
- What additional questions should you ask the client?

Nanette telephones the client the next day. The client's vocal quality sounds worse than the day before, and when asked about the medications the client says to talk about something else.

- What do you think is going on with the client's medications?
- Where might you find out more information about the medications?

Nanette decides to contact the health plan to find out if any recent claims were paid for the client's medication. The health insurance nurse says that the medication was discontinued from the health plan's formulary and coverage for the medication ended the previous month.

- What should you do now?
- What should you say to the health insurance nurse?

Nanette contacts the client again and explains knowing about the medication being discontinued from coverage. The client admits to rationing the few doses of the remaining medication but does not want to make an appointment to see the doctor because of the high copayments.

- What would you like to do at this time?
- Who should you contact first: the health plan or the client's physician/health care provider?

Nanette discusses the client's medication issue with the health care provider's nurse. The client is mailed a prescription for a comparable medication that is covered by the health plan's medication coverage. When Nanette contacts the client in a few days, the client's vocal quality is much improved.

- As a fellow telephonic nurse, do you feel that Nanette did the right thing?
- What else might you consider doing to help this client prevent this situation in the future?

KEY POINTS

- Neurologic and sensory disorders can be extremely challenging for the client. Most of these disorders do not improve, and the client has to make lifelong adjustments to perform activities of daily living.
- Be sure to take your time when assessing these clients. Listen to the terms the client uses to describe the disorder.
- Always support the physician/health care provider's plan of care. Clients may feel desperate and want to try another treatment approach. Strongly encourage clients to discuss these approaches with their physician/health care provider before proceeding. Clients may be prescribed medications that could cause adverse effects if taken with herb or vitamin supplements.
- At first, the client may be skeptical regarding the telephonic care calls. Explain the purpose as helping to prevent future hospitalizations or acute exacerbations.

BIBLIOGRAPHY

D'Amico, D., & Barbarito, C. (2012). *Health and physical assessment in nursing* (2nd ed.). Upper Saddle River, NJ: Pearson.

Lemone, P. (2015). *Medical-surgical nursing* (6th ed.). Upper Saddle River, NJ: Pearson.

Pearson Education. (2015). *Nursing: A Concept-based approach to learning* (2nd ed., Vol. 2). Upper Saddle River, NJ: Author.

CHAPTER 18

Disorders of the Genitourinary System

LEARNING OUTCOMES

Upon completion of this chapter, the nurse will:

1. Summarize the different disorders of the genitourinary system
2. Examine approaches to assess different disorders of the genitourinary system
3. Determine approaches that can be used for more than one genitourinary system disorder

GENITOURINARY SYSTEM DISORDERS

Disorders within the genitourinary system can be acute, chronic, or an adverse effect caused by a medication or other health problem. The disorders that would be the most appropriate for telephonic care include:

- Acute renal failure (recovery from)
- Chronic renal failure
- Kidney stones
- Urinary tract infection
- Prostatitis
- Benign prostatic hyperplasia (BPH)
- Prostate cancer
- Benign breast disease
- Breast cancer

Disorders that "might come up" in the course of a conversation that would not necessarily be considered a reason for disease management include:

- Urinary incontinence
- Erectile dysfunction
- Menstrual difficulties
- Menopausal difficulties

ASSESSING DISORDERS OF THE GENITOURINARY SYSTEM

Remember that the client has been diagnosed with a genitourinary system problem. The assessment should focus on the client's current status and if there have been any changes in symptoms.

Health Problem	Changes
Acute renal failure	When were you told you had a kidney problem?
	What caused it, such as: ● An injury? ● Kidney stone? ● Infection?
	How are you feeling right now?
	Has your urine output returned to the amount prior to the problem?
	What medicines have you been taking for the problem?
	When are you supposed to see your doctor or health care provider again for the kidney problem?
	For what reasons have you been directed by your doctor or health care provider to seek additional medical care because of the kidney problem?
Chronic renal failure	When were you told that you have chronic kidney problems?
	What treatment are you having? ● Peritoneal dialysis? ● Hemodialysis?

(continued)

(*continued*)

Health Problem	Changes
	(If hemodialysis) On which arm is your fistula for the treatments?
	How does the skin over the fistula look?
	Can you feel anything when you touch the skin over the fistula like a buzzing or vibration?
	When do you have treatments, such as: • Monday, Wednesday, and Friday? • Tuesday, Thursday, and Saturday?
	(If peritoneal dialysis) Do you do the treatments at home or at the kidney center? How often do you have treatments? Are you having any problems, such as: • Blood in the drainage? • Cloudy drainage? • Abdominal pain? • Fever?
	What medicine are you taking because of the kidney failure? • Are you taking the medicine as prescribed? • Are you having any side effects from the medicine? • Are you receiving a medicine that is injected every week to 10 days?
	What diet changes have you had to make because of the kidney failure, such as: • Reduce dairy products? • Avoid foods high in potassium?
	Are you considering or being considered for a kidney transplant? • If so, what have you been told about the transplant?
	When are you supposed to see your doctor or health care provider again for the kidney problem?
	For what reasons have you been directed by your doctor or health care provider to seek additional medical care because of the kidney problem?

(*continued*)

(continued)

Health Problem	Changes
Kidney stones (renal calculi)	When were you told that you have kidney stones?
	What symptoms are you having right now, such as: • Flank pain? • Groin pain? • Blood in the urine?
	What treatment are you having/had for the kidney stones? • Lithotripsy? • Medication?
	Have you been directed to strain your urine? If so, what has been strained out?
	Have you been directed to make dietary or fluid intake changes? If so, what changes have you made? • Reduce dairy? • Increased fluid?
	When are you supposed to see your doctor or health care provider again for the kidney stones?
	For what reasons have you been directed by your doctor or health care provider to seek additional medical care because of the kidney stones?
Urinary tract infection	When were you told that you have a urinary tract infection?
	What symptoms are you having right now, such as: • Burning with urination? • Blood in the urine? • Low-grade fever?
	What medicine are you taking for the infection, such as: • Antibiotics? • Antispasmodics?
	What information were you told about the medicine, such as: • Take the full course of the antibiotics even if the symptoms of the infection go away

(continued)

(continued)

Health Problem	Changes
	How often do you take the medicine for the bladder spasms? Is the medication helping?
	What other information were you told to help prevent future infections, such as: • Appropriate cleansing after toileting? • Increasing the intake of oral fluids? • Wearing breathable clothing? • Voiding after intercourse? • Not ignoring the urge to void? • Avoiding tub baths?
	When are you supposed to see your doctor or health care provider again for the infection?
	For what reasons have you been directed by your doctor or health care provider to seek additional medical care because of the infection?
Prostatitis	When were you told that you have prostatitis?
	Is this the first time that you have had the problem or have you had it before?
	What symptoms are you having right now, such as: • Low-back pain? • Discomfort with sitting? • Weak urinary stream? • Pain with ejaculation?
	What medicine are you taking for the prostatitis, such as: • Antibiotics? • Nonsteroidal anti-inflammatory agents?
	What else have you been directed to do to help with the problem, such as: • Avoid sitting for long periods of time? • Taking a warm tub bath?
	When are you supposed to see your doctor or health care provider again for the problem?
	For what reasons have you been directed by your doctor or health care provider to seek additional medical care because of the problem?

(continued)

(*continued*)

Health Problem	Changes
Benign prostatic hyperplasia (BPH)	When were you told that you have BPH?
	What tests did you have done? • Digital exam? • Blood tests? • Urine tests? • Biopsy?
	What symptoms are you having right now, such as: • Urinary frequency? • Dribbling?
	What medicine are you taking for the BPH? • Are you taking the medicines prescribed? • Have you noticed if the medicine is helping?
	Were you or are you using anything else for the symptoms, such as: • Saw palmetto? • Echinacea?
	Are you going to have/had surgery for the problem? • When will it be done? (Postoperative: When was it done?) • What was done? • How are you feeling right now?
	When are you supposed to see your doctor/health care provider again for the BPH?
	For what reasons have you been directed by your doctor/health care provider to seek additional medical care because of the BPH?
Prostate cancer	When were you told that you have prostate cancer?
	What tests did you have done, such as: • Blood test (prostate-specific antigen [PSA])? • Biopsy? • Digital examination?

(*continued*)

(continued)

Health Problem	Changes
	What symptoms are you having right now, such as: • Pain with urination? • Frequency? • Blood in the urine? • Bone or joint pain? • Lower extremity weakness? • Weight loss? • Fatigue?
	What treatment are you having for the prostate cancer, such as: • Surgery? • Medication? • Radiation? • Watch and wait?
	When are you supposed to see your doctor/ health care provider again for the prostate cancer?
	For what reasons have you been directed by your doctor/health care provider to seek additional medical care because of the prostate cancer?
Benign breast disease	When were you told that you have a breast condition?
	What were you told that you have?
	What symptoms are you having right now, such as: • Breast pain? • Nipple discharge?
	What have you been directed to do to help with the breast condition, such as: • Wearing a well-fitted bra? • Avoiding coffee, tea, cola, and chocolate? • Using over-the-counter pain medication? • Applying heat/cold?
	When are you supposed to see your doctor/ health care provider again for the breast condition?

(continued)

(*continued*)

Health Problem	Changes
	For what reasons have you been directed by your doctor/health care provider to seek additional medical care because of the breast condition?
Breast cancer	When were you told that you have breast cancer?
	When was your last mammogram?
	When was the biopsy done?
	What were you told when you received the results of the biopsy?

	What treatment are you having/going to have:
	• Chemotherapy:
	  ▪ When will/did this start?
	  ▪ How many treatments/how many weeks?
	• Radiation:
	  ▪ When will/did this start?
	  ▪ How many treatments/how many weeks?
	• Surgery:
	  ▪ When will this be/was this done?
	  ▪ What type will be/was done (remove the entire breast, remove a portion of the breast)?

	What information were you given about the treatments, such as: • Potential for nausea and hair loss with chemotherapy? • Skin care for radiation treatments? • Risk for arm swelling (lymphedema) after breast surgery?
	How are you feeling right now? (The client with breast cancer can have many psychosocial issues. The best approach would be to ask: What can I do to help you right now?)
	When are you supposed to see your doctor/health care provider again?
	For what reasons have you been directed by your doctor/health care provider to seek additional medical care?

ADDITIONAL DISORDERS

It is unlikely that a client will be enrolled in a disease management program for problems with urinary incontinence, menstruation, menopause, or erectile dysfunction; however, these problems may be identified during the course of a regular care call.

Problem	Questions
Urinary incontinence	Assess when the problem started
	Assess when the problem occurs: • Stress: occurs when sneezing, coughing • Urge: loss of urine with a strong urge to void • Overflow: bladder does not empty and excess urine leaks out • Functional: cannot get to the bathroom in time because of physical problem
	Assess the frequency that this occurs
	Assess what has been done about it: • Wearing protection • Bathing more frequently • Voiding schedule
	Assess if medication has been prescribed and the effectiveness of the medication
	Encourage to adhere to prescribed treatment plan or seek medical attention for any new onset of symptoms.
Erectile dysfunction	Assess for length of time the problem has been occurring
	Assess if the problem has been discussed with a health care professional
	Assess if the problem can be associated with taking a newly prescribed medication (such as antihypertensives, other cardiac medications) or disease process (diabetes)
	Suggest to discuss the problem with a health care professional

(continued)

(*continued*)

Problem	Questions
Menstrual difficulties	Assess for the type of difficulty: ● Cramping ● Large blood flow ● Clotting ● Bleeding between menstrual cycles
	Assess for the length of time the problem has been occurring
	Assess for what has been done to help with the problem: ● Applying heat (cramps) ● Changing diet (cramps) ● Increasing activity (cramps) ● Resting (large blood flow/clotting)
	Suggest discussing the problem with a health care professional
Menopausal difficulties	Assess for the type of difficulty: ● Hot flashes ● Night sweats ● Insomnia ● Painful urination ● Painful intercourse
	Assess for the length of time the problem has been occurring
	Assess for what has been done to help with the problem: ● Exercise ● Daily calcium intake ● Water-soluble lubricant ● Increased fluid intake ● Wearing breathable clothing ● Complementary/alternative therapies or supplements
	Suggest to discuss the problem with a health care professional

SUGGESTIONS FOR GENITOURINARY DISORDERS

● Use the same terminology that the client uses to describe the problem.
● Always ask how the patient/client is feeling right now.

● Genitourinary disorders can adversely affect activities of daily living. The patient may restrict leaving the home and change routine activities because of the fear of becoming incontinent during an inopportune time. Assess how the problem has affected regular activities.

● Remember that talking about this body system and problems can cause the patient embarrassment. Keep the conversation "matter of fact" and do not proceed if the patient refuses to discuss any problems further.

● Ask about the prescribed treatment for a health problem and reinforce the treatment. Do not recommend a complementary or alternative therapy. If asked about something that is not mainstream treatment, encourage the patient to discuss the approach with the health care professional.

PRACTICE EXERCISES

Read the following client situations and determine:

● Which questions to ask
● What the client might be experiencing
● Whether the situation requires the client to contact the doctor or health care provider

1. A client recovering from a kidney infection asks why the urine has blood in it.
2. During a care call, a client recovering from acute renal failure asks if it is normal to not have to urinate for over 24 hours.
3. A client with a history of renal stones is experiencing new back and groin pain.
4. While assessing another body system, an older client asks if the heart problem is causing urinary incontinence.
5. A client being treated for a urinary tract infection asks how long antibiotics can be saved.
6. A client with prostatitis says that laying down makes the pain more bearable.
7. A client in the diabetes management program says that skipping doses of medications helps with the hot flashes from menopause.
8. A client receiving radiation for prostate cancer asks if the back and bone pain means that the disease is being cured.

9. A young adult client in a wellness program says that the only thing that helps with menstrual cramps is alcohol.
10. Before ending a care call, a client with chronic renal failure asks what can be done to stop the bleeding from the fistula site.

CASE STUDY

Yvette, a telephonic nurse for a disease management company, is scheduled to contact several clients with chronic urinary conditions. During the first call, the male client with BPH says he doesn't want to talk about the problem.

- What would you do?
- What could you say to encourage the client to talk about the problem without embarrassment?

The next client is receiving radiation treatments for prostate cancer and says that he is having problems washing the marks off of his skin.

- What should you say to this client?
- What additional teaching might this client need?

After lunch Yvette is to contact clients with a variety of female genitourinary disorders. The first client is being treated for breast cancer and is experiencing extreme nausea and vomiting from the chemotherapy.

- What should you suggest to this client?
- What additional information would be helpful to gather from this client?

Prior to leaving for the day, Yvette takes an incoming call from a client who is distraught. The client has not been able to sleep "for days" because of extreme hot flashes during the night.

- What additional information should you obtain from this client?
- What should you suggest to this client?

KEY POINTS

- Unless a patient/client is diagnosed with a genitourinary disorder, most issues with this body system will occur with another health problem.
- Discussing this body system can be embarrassing to many people.
- Urinary incontinence is not a normal expected age-related change. Patients/clients experiencing this health problem should discuss it with their health care professional.
- Pain and blood in the urine are not normal body findings. Encourage the patient/client to seek medical attention if these occur.

BIBLIOGRAPHY

D'Amico, D., & Barbarito, C. (2012). *Health and physical assessment in nursing* (2nd ed.). Upper Saddle River, NJ: Pearson.

Lemone, P. (2015). *Medical-surgical nursing* (6th ed.). Upper Saddle River, NJ: Pearson.

Pearson Education. (2015). *Nursing: A concept-based approach to learning* (2nd ed., Vol. 2). Upper Saddle River, NJ: Author.

CHAPTER 19

The Patient/Client With Diabetes Mellitus

LEARNING OUTCOMES

Upon completion of this chapter, the nurse will:

1. Summarize the difference between type 1 and type 2 diabetes mellitus
2. Examine approaches to assess diabetes mellitus
3. Determine strategies to aid the patient/client with diabetes mellitus

TYPES OF DIABETES MELLITUS

A complete review of diabetes mellitus is beyond the intention of this text. Rather, a brief review of the types of diabetes will be provided along with anticipated or expected effects if the disease is not adequately managed.

Type 1 diabetes mellitus is caused by destruction of the beta cells (islets of Langerhans) in the liver. The body does not produce insulin, a hormone for which a continuous supply is required. At one point, it was believed that type 1 diabetes mellitus was a disease of childhood. Through ongoing research, it was discovered that anyone at any age can develop this type of diabetes.

Type 2 diabetes mellitus is caused by insulin resistance. The body has been making insulin in response to dietary intake that, over time, causes the beta cells to become fatigued. In addition, the body ceases to recognize or use available insulin in the tissues. This form of the disease is considered the most prevalent and can also occur at any age. In the past, type 2 diabetes mellitus occurred most often in middle age but is increasingly being diagnosed in preadolescent children.

COMPLICATIONS

The major complication of type 1 diabetes mellitus is diabetic ketoacidosis (DKA), whereas the major complication for type 2 diabetes mellitus is hyperosmolar hyperglycemic state (HHS). In both conditions, the blood glucose levels are wildly elevated and cause tremendous adverse effects. Additional manifestations of these complications are as follows:

Manifestations of DKA	Manifestations of HHS
Dehydration ● Weakness ● Malaise ● Hypotension ● Dry mucous membranes	Dehydration ● Extreme thirst ● Altered level of consciousness
Ketosis ● Nausea and vomiting ● Ketone breath odor	Excessive urine output
Abdominal pain	Neurologic deficits
Kussmaul's respirations	Lactic acidosis

Further complications of diabetes mellitus are categorized as being either macrovascular or microvascular. Macrovascular complications include:

● Coronary artery disease
● Hypertension
● Stroke
● Peripheral vascular disease

And microvascular complications are:

● Retinopathy
● Nephropathy
● Neuropathy

Even though diabetes affects all body organs, it causes the most harm to the blood vessels, the eyes, the kidneys, and peripheral nerves.

It is because of these complications that individuals with either type of the disease should be counseled to have:

- Routine eye examinations
- Annual assessment of urine albumin levels
- Routine assessment of blood pressure
- Frequent examinations of the feet

GENERAL TELEPHONIC CARE NEEDS

One of the first telephonic disease management programs was for diabetes, and these programs continue today. It has been found that, for people with diabetes, telephonic care reduces the onset of macro- and microcomplications and subsequent hospitalizations.

The purpose of contacting people in these programs is to reinforce their prescribed treatment plan. In general, the major categories when providing care are:

- Self-monitoring
- Medications
- Nutritional intake
- Activity/exercise
- Diagnostic evaluation
- Preventive actions

Self-Monitoring

Patients/clients are instructed to perform capillary blood glucose testing at various times. As a telephonic nurse, you need to first find out how frequently the testing is being done. Oftentimes, clients receive the monitors as a service from different pharmaceutical companies; however, the supplies to use the monitors (strips, reagent liquid) can be costly. Before encouraging a client to increase capillary testing, listen to how the client responds to the expected frequency. For example, if the client says "those strips are so expensive so I only test once in the morning," encouraging the client to increase the frequency of the testing will not be productive.

Urine testing for ketones and glucose may be done by some clients with type 1 diabetes mellitus; however, it is not widely used for those with type 2.

Medications

At one point, insulin was reserved to treat individuals with type 1 diabetes mellitus, and oral agents were used to treat those with type 2 of the disease. This is not the case anymore. Although the only treatment for type 1 diabetes mellitus is insulin, those with type 2 may be treated with either oral agents, insulin, or both.

Insulin

When assessing medications, be sure to correctly document the type of insulin being used and the amount in units. Your care regarding insulin use should focus on:

- Ability to fill syringes
- Ability to self-administer doses
- Identification of appropriate injection sites
- Avoidance of hypertrophy or atrophy of subcutaneous tissue
- Appropriate timing of injections (based on the type of insulin used)

Oral Agents

New oral agents to treat type 2 diabetes mellitus are constantly being developed. The most recent classifications for these medications with examples are:

- Sulfonylureas
  - Glipizide (Glucotrol)
  - Glyburide (DiaBeta, Micronase)
  - Glimepiride (Amaryl)

- Biguanides
  - Metformin (Glucophage)

- Alpha-glucoside inhibitors
  - Acarbose (Precose)
  - Miglitol (Glyset)

- Meglitinides
  - Repaglinide (Prandin)

- DPP-4 inhibitors
  - Sitagliptin (Januvia)

- Synthetic amylin hormone
  - Pramlintide (Symtin)

Assessing current medications includes the name, dose, and frequency being taken.

Nonspecified Medication

One noninsulin medication used to treat type 2 diabetes mellitus is injected; however, it is not insulin—it is the incretin mimetic exenatide (Byetta). It is injected before the morning and evening meals; never after a meal.

Nutritional Intake

For some clients with diabetes, dietary management can be the most challenging aspect of self-care. Many years ago, people with diabetes were handed a diet to follow in order to control blood glucose levels. As research in the disease progressed, the philosophy of following a strict diet has decreased to be replaced with eating plans that support the client's preferences while controlling the intake of carbohydrates.

Weight management is often included in the treatment plan for those with type 2 diabetes mellitus. At times, losing a predetermined percentage of body weight has helped reduce the need for medication to treat the disorder. This approach is not successful for all clients with the disease.

A client with this disorder might ask you to "send a diet" to follow to help control blood glucose levels. Because this is rarely if ever done, the client may benefit from discussing meal planning with a nutritionist or dietitian. Should a client be provided with an eating plan from a health care provider, ask the client to tell you the daily calorie intake and number of carbohydrate servings per day. This information is helpful to have available for future care calls.

Activity and Exercise

Individuals with diabetes are encouraged to maintain and often increase their activity level. Inactivity has been found to contribute to increased body weight and the onset of type 2 diabetes mellitus. Before promoting any particular physical activity, assess the patient/client for current activity status. There are many online tools that subdivide activity status into categories such as sedentary, light activity, moderate, and heavy activity. A good starting point might be to ask what type of employment the client engages in. Then you can ask what type of physical activity the client routinely participates in, such as walking the dog every morning and evening, swimming at the local health facility, or playing tennis or golf on the weekends. You might find that some older clients spend the vast majority of the day sitting. For these individuals, exercise might be walking up and down the steps in the home several times a day or walking to the mailbox. Another suggestion might be to walk in a grocery store or shopping mall if inclement weather is a factor. Not every client is able or capable of engaging in an outdoor walking program. And, depending on where the client lives and socioeconomic status, joining a health facility or club may not be an option.

Remember that an activity or exercise program should not be encouraged unless it is supported by the health care provider. The client will most likely state that "my doctor told me to get more exercise" or "I was told I have to move more if I expect to lose weight." These comments indicate that the health care provider has discussed physical activity with the client.

Diagnostic Evaluation

Although the client may be measuring capillary blood glucose values daily, the hemoglobin A1c blood test is considered the gold standard when evaluating the success of glycemic control. This test determines the average blood glucose levels over the previous 6 to 12 weeks and is typically measured every 3 months. Each client's goal for the hemoglobin A1c will be determined by the health care provider.

Additional tests will most likely be prescribed to determine the development or presence of macro- or microcomplications. These diagnostic tests include:

- Urine albumin level
- Serum blood urea nitrogen
- Serum creatinine
- Lipid panel
- Electrocardiogram

You may or may not automatically receive the results of these tests within the client's medical record so asking if the client has received the blood/urine results would be an appropriate discussion. Then depending on the results, you can alter the content of your care call accordingly.

Clients with diabetes should be encouraged to have an annual eye examination, regardless of the client's age. The only way to determine if glycemic control is affecting the vasculature of the eyes is to have routine ophthalmologic evaluations. This action cannot be emphasized enough with the client.

Preventive Actions

There are a number of actions that a client can take to help reduce or prevent the development of complications from diabetes. These actions include:

- Routine dental examinations
- Daily foot assessment
- Wearing properly fitting footwear at all times
- Getting adequate rest/sleep
- Keeping routine health care provider appointments
- Smoking cessation

Routine Dental Examinations

Clients may ask what the teeth have to do with diabetes. Because elevated blood glucose levels affect every body tissue, there is a risk for the development of periodontal disease in these clients. Ensuring that the gums and teeth are healthy by routine examinations and teeth cleaning reduces this risk.

Daily Foot Assessment

Clients with diabetes are prone to developing peripheral neuropathy, especially of the feet. Television commercials advertising medication for this health problem often call this disorder "diabetic nerve pain" so clients may use this same terminology. Manifestations of this type of nerve pain include numbness, tingling, and sharp pain. Because of the change in sensory status of the feet, clients with diabetes are prone to developing foot wounds. It is essential to remind these clients to look at the bottom of the feet every day. If the client is unable to physically pick up the foot to look at the skin integrity, suggest that a mirror be placed on the floor or against the wall to be used to see the bottom of the foot.

Wearing Properly Fitting Footwear at All Times

Although it might sound like common sense, some people do not wear shoes or any footwear when in the home or walking out of doors. For the person with diabetes, this could be a deadly action. Individuals with this disorder should also be reminded that shoes should have enough room at the toes and should fit well but not rub at the heel. And, if shopping for new shoes, the best time would be at the end of the day when the feet are at their maximum size. Shoes purchased early in the day may become progressively tighter if worn throughout the entire day. For a person with diabetes, tight shoes can lead to blisters, ulcers, and, unfortunately, wounds.

Getting Adequate Rest and Sleep

Getting adequate rest does not mean that the person with diabetes should take frequent naps and schedule rest periods between activities. This means that if the person is feeling tired or fatigued, rest should be considered.

Insufficient sleep can increase the body's levels of cortisol, the stress hormone. Increasing these levels adversely affects blood glucose, causing the level to rise. Actions to reduce stress cannot be emphasized enough with these clients.

Keeping Routine Health Care Provider Appointments

A client with diabetes should expect to see the health care provider every 3 to 6 months. Blood work will be completed along with additional testing as required and based on the results of the examination. Medication may be changed or doses adjusted.

When preparing to see the health care provider, clients should be reminded to take off their shoes and socks so that the feet can be examined. This should be done for every appointment. The health care provider may use a tool with a monofilament to gently touch areas on the bottom and top of the foot, assessing the sensory status and ultimately the integrity of the peripheral nerves.

Smoking Cessation

Cigarette smoking has been identified as a culprit for many cardiovascular diseases, and it negatively affects the person with diabetes as well. In diabetes, the blood vessels are harmed by uncontrolled blood glucose levels. When the chemicals and nicotine from cigarette smoke are added, these blood vessels are at risk for additional harm. Asking the client about current smoking behavior is essential. Then information about smoking cessation activities can be offered as appropriate.

Acute Illnesses

Clients with diabetes who experience an acute illness such as the flu should be reminded to take medication as prescribed even if their dietary intake is less than what is usually ingested. When acutely ill the body is stressed. Cortisol levels will be affected, and blood glucose levels may rise. If medication is taken as prescribed, the body will not be additionally stressed with hyperglycemia. Always encourage the patient/client with diabetes to discuss specific medication treatment approaches for an acute illness with the health care provider.

Acute Hypoglycemia

Even the person who tightly controls the blood glucose level can experience episodes of hypoglycemia. A change in weather, unplanned for activity or exercise, or skipping a meal or snack can cause the blood glucose level to plummet. Clients with diabetes should be reminded to keep a source of rapid-acting glucose available at all times. For some, this might be glucose tablets. Others may keep a tube of icing.

Clients should be asked to describe the symptoms of a low blood glucose level and be reminded to never ignore these symptoms. Over time, if these symptoms are ignored and the falling blood glucose level is not addressed, the body may cease to send these signals. Losing these signals can lead to "hypoglycemia unawareness." This means that the person with diabetes may not experience symptoms of hypoglycemia until the blood glucose level is dangerously low. Should this occur, a rapid acting source of glucose, such as icing, would be ideal. The client will not be able to safely swallow glucose tables or liquids. Icing can be placed under the tongue or along the cheek for rapid absorption into the bloodstream.

For the client treating acute hypoglycemia at home, there is a process called "15 every 15" that can be used. This means that once a low blood glucose level is obtained, 15 g of a carbohydrate should be ingested and recheck the blood glucose level in 15 minutes. If the level has not increased, another 15 g of carbohydrate should be ingested followed by another blood glucose level check in 15 minutes. This is to be repeated until the symptoms subside and the blood glucose level returns to a normal level.

Acute hypoglycemia can also occur after exercise. For this reason, people with diabetes should be reminded to ingest 15 g of carbohydrates before exercising and to have an additional source of glucose to ingest afterward.

SPECIAL SITUATION

The primary manifestations of diabetes are polyuria, polyphagia, and polydipsia. Even in the presence of polyphagia, the person with undiagnosed and untreated type 1 diabetes mellitus will lose weight. Once the disease is diagnosed and medication treatment started, body weight should stabilize. For most people, this is a desired effect; however, an adolescent or young adult may not agree.

For some adolescents and young adults, weight loss is welcomed regardless of the detrimental effects to the body. Long-term effects may not mean much to a younger person now; however, having a thinner body today is a bonus. These clients might be particularly challenging when discussing medication adherence during a telephonic care call.

Suggestions to increase medication adherence include:

- Explain the effects of extended hyperglycemia on the eyes, kidneys, heart, and nerve endings.
- Discuss the potential for foot wounds and other organ damage.
- Positively reinforce efforts when taking medication as prescribed.

Clients within this age population may also be at the mercy of peer pressure and may not want to have to do something that is "different" from friends. Friends are not having to check blood glucose levels several times a day, self-administer injections, or see the school nurse every few days for a diabetes-related health issue. For these clients, alternative insulin-providing devices such as the pump might be the preferred medication administration route. The client should be encouraged to discuss alternative avenues to ensure medication adherence with the health care provider.

CARE CALLS

Now that you are adequately armed with all of this information to provide care to a client with diabetes, how should the calls proceed? The following provides an example of a series of calls for the client with diabetes.

Calls	Content
First call (Some organizations refer to this call as the welcome call or engagement call and is usually the longest of the care calls)	• Review the purpose of the program • Obtain client willingness to participate in routine care calls • Validate demographic information • Obtain best day and time for future calls • Establish frequency of future calls • Obtain baseline medication and laboratory data from the client • Ask if there is anything in particular with which the client is having an issue or desires additional information • End the call with an estimated day/time for the next call
Second call (Some organizations might refer to this as a routine care call or follow-up call)	• Reinforce anything discussed from the welcome/engagement call • Ask if there is anything in particular with which the client is having an issue or desires addition information. Address this need first. • Methodically begin going through aspects of the client's care needs. For some, this might be medication adherence or weight management.

(continued)

(continued)

Calls	Content
	For others, this might mean keeping scheduled health care provider appointments or approaches to reduce carbohydrate intake to control blood glucose levels. • Document the content discussed and the client's response during the call • End the call with an estimated day/time for the next call
Third and subsequent calls	• Reinforce anything discussed from the previous call • Ask if there is anything in particular with which the client is having an issue or desires addition information. Address this need first. • Continue with discussing aspects of the client's care needs. Use this text as a guide, keeping in mind the categories of: ▪ Medication ▪ Activity/exercise ▪ Weight management ▪ Diagnostic tests ▪ Prevention of complications ▪ Foot care ▪ Keeping appointments with the health care provider ▪ Self-care when ill ▪ Self-treatment for acute hypoglycemia ▪ Smoking behavior • Always provide positive reinforcement for any changes made that positively impact the client's self-management of the disease process

DISEASE MANAGEMENT PROGRAM EXPECTATIONS

Without a doubt, nurses know how to instruct and what to include when discussing a chronic disease such as diabetes mellitus with a client. But at times, an organization or health plan may want specific "things" discussed with the clients in these programs. For example, a disease management program might want to emphasize the importance of clients having an annual influenza vaccination in the autumn of the year. You will need to include this information when providing care calls to the clients during this time period. Other examples of information that may be required by the organization or health plan include:

- Date of last eye examination
- Date of electrocardiogram
- Date of next scheduled health care provider appointment

Another expectation might be for the organization or health plan to expect you to send the client specific teaching tools. Depending on the sophistication of the documentation system and the client, these tools may be sent via e-mail or hard copy through the mail system. Regardless of the method used, you will most likely be expected to document the tool sent, the date, and then any follow-up provided once the client has had a chance to review the material. Expect the selection, mailing, and follow-up of mailed items to continue through the life of the client's participation in the program.

KEY POINTS: WRAPPING IT ALL UP

- Because the incidence of diabetes mellitus has been incrementally increasing over the years and can cause life-altering and potentially life-threatening adverse effects, diabetes disease management programs are prevalent.
- Even though there are two types of the disease, the care call needs are generally the same.
- Realize that the calls to these patients/clients will span over months and possibly years.
- Keep the medication listing and most recent diagnostic data as current as possible. This means asking if the patient/client has had any changes to medications since the last care call or if any new laboratory values were provided during the last health care provider examination.
- Always ask if the patient/client has any questions or needs first before discussing an aspect of self-care.
- For challenging situations, brainstorm approaches with the patient/client. This helps gain acceptance and adherence.
- Remember to applaud any success that the patient/client demonstrates. This might mean cheering for the client who has never

walked to the mailbox but has been doing that activity every day for 2 weeks. Or the client who has replaced sugary beverages with diet soda. Every change, regardless of the magnitude, can have long-term positive effects to the client's health.

● Enjoy the calls and look forward to "checking-in" with your patients/clients. In time, the clients will also look forward to the calls and may even contact you to report a major change or success!

BIBLIOGRAPHY

Lemone, P. (2015). *Medical-surgical nursing* (6th ed.). Upper Saddle River, NJ: Pearson.

Pearson Education. (2015). *Nursing: A concept-based approach to learning* (2nd ed., Vol. 2). Upper Saddle River, NJ: Author.

Van Leeuwen, A. W., & Bladh, M. L. (2015). *Comprehensive handbook of laboratory & diagnostic tests with nursing implications* (6th ed.). Philadelphia, PA: F. A. Davis.

Wilson, B. A., Shannon, M. T., & Shields, K. M. (2015). *Pearson nurse's drug guide 2016*. Upper Saddle River, NJ: Pearson.

CHAPTER 20

The Patient/Client With HIV/AIDS

LEARNING OUTCOMES

Upon completion of this chapter, the nurse will:

1. Summarize the pathophysiology of HIV/AIDS
2. Examine approaches to assess the patient/client with HIV/AIDS
3. Determine strategies to aid the patient/client with HIV/AIDS

PATHOPHYSIOLOGY REVIEW OF HIV/AIDS

HIV is a retrovirus that is transmitted through blood and body fluids. It was first diagnosed in 1984 after the discovery of a specific antigen–antibody complex. A constellation of body changes occurs when the HIV enters the body:

- Virus attacks one type of cell called T lymphocytes
- Virus duplicates through normal cell division
- T lymphocytes become inactivated and immunity is compromised

Manifestations of HIV can range from no symptoms to severe immune system collapse. When first infected, the person may experience:

- Fever
- Body aches and pains
- Sore throat
- Headache
- Nausea/vomiting
- Rash

These manifestations are similar to many other infections and disease processes, which makes it difficult to diagnose at first. And, it takes weeks to months for the body to develop antibodies to the virus. Even so, the person is extremely contagious during this time.

A person learns of having HIV through voluntary testing. A person might believe an exposure to body fluid or blood occurred through intimacy and asks for testing to be done. Or, a health care professional might have accidentally received a needle stick and testing is part of the postexposure care. Another way HIV testing maybe completed is if a person is planning to store blood for auto-transfusion for an upcoming surgery or is participating as a blood donor.

Once considered an immediate death sentence, people with HIV can live many healthy years if medication treatment is initiated and continued without interruption. Should there be a change in the person's health status or medication treatment ceases to be effective, AIDS can develop. The diagnosis of AIDS is dire because the T lymphocyte levels are dangerously low and the person can develop an array of opportunistic infections.

CHALLENGES

Disease management programs created for HIV/AIDS started in the mid to late 1990s and were sponsored by state and federal programs through Medicaid. Several states have published the results and successes of these programs; however, there is still much to be accomplished.

One of the major issues when working with this population is confidentiality. The results of an HIV/AIDS test are confidential, and there needs to be controls built in so that patient/client confidentiality is not breached.

States with HIV/AIDS Medicaid programs enroll individuals with the illness into their disease management program. The individual receives written communication about being enrolled and has an opportunity to accept enrollment or decline. There is no penalty for choosing to decline; however, the major benefit for participating is an improvement in the person's health. The states with these programs have to guarantee that all communication complies with the Health Insurance Portability and Accountability Act (HIPAA) privacy standards.

BENEFITS

Besides enhancing the number of healthy years living with HIV and preventing the development of AIDS, specific advantages of using telephonic disease management for this client population includes reducing the number of:

- Sexually transmitted infections (STIs)
- Hepatitis B infections
- Tuberculosis infections

PRIMARY CARE FOCUS

The focus when providing telephonic care to a person with HIV is not to discuss the way in which the infection was obtained. Care calls should focus on:

- Current health status
- Any changes in symptoms
- Any new manifestations
- Adherence to prescribed medication regimen
- Any adverse effects of medications

Current Health Status

Ideally, the person with HIV would not be aware of having an illness. Others with the disorder may experience one or more swollen lymph nodes.

Changes in Symptoms

Any changes in symptoms need to be further investigated and substantiated with a T lymphocyte cell count (CD4 T-cell count). These changes can include:

- Malaise
- Persistent fever
- Fatigue

- Weight loss
- Night sweats
- Rash

The patient might also experience neurologic symptoms such as changes in motor and sensory function. These changes may be due to the effects of the virus on the nerve endings or indicate that the disease is progressing.

New Manifestations

New manifestations would most likely be associated with the development of opportunistic infections. The development of these infections is an indication that the patient is progressing into AIDS and include:

- Pneumocystis pneumonia
- Tuberculosis
- Herpes virus
- Herpes zoster
- Toxoplasma parasitic infections
- Protozoan infections of the gastrointestinal tract
- *Candida albicans*
- Pelvic inflammatory disease

The patient may also develop what are considered secondary cancers. The most prominent cancers seen in AIDS include:

- Kaposi's sarcoma
- Lymphoma
- Cervical cancer

And other disease processes that may develop in the client with AIDS are:

- Coronary heart disease
- Liver disease
- Nephropathy

Adherence to Prescribed Medication Regimen

The medication regimen for patients with HIV/AIDS is complicated. There are currently six drug classifications of antiretroviral medications used to treat the disease:

- CCR5 antagonists
- Fusion inhibitors
- Integrase strand transfer inhibitors
- Non-nucleoside reverse transcriptase inhibitors
- Nucleoside reverse transcriptase inhibitors
- Protease inhibitors

The current protocol is for a patient to take three of the medications spanning at least two of the different drug classifications. The medications are selected according to T lymphocyte blood levels and other symptoms. For maximum effectiveness, the medications should not be stopped or interrupted at any time. If any medication is to be discontinued, the dosage should be tapered.

Adverse Effects of Medications

Antiretroviral medications are expensive and can cause extreme adverse effects. These issues contribute to the poor levels of medication adherence.

Zidovudine (AZT) was the first antiretroviral drug developed. The major adverse effects of this nucleoside reverse transcriptase inhibitor are nausea and vomiting. Other antiretroviral medication should be taken with food to avoid gastrointestinal irritation. Protease inhibitors cause metabolic changes such as diabetes mellitus and changes in cholesterol and triglyceride levels. Alteration in the composition and distribution of body fat also occurs with this medication, specifically abdominal obesity and wasting of the extremities.

Other issues with medications to treat HIV/AIDS include the timing of medications, if the dose needs to be taken on an empty stomach or with a meal, and swallowing the dose whole or chewing a tablet.

ASSESSING THE PATIENT/CLIENT WITH HIV/AIDS

The patient/client should have received a letter or other form of communication about being enrolled in the program prior to you making the first call. The letter should explain the purpose of the program and allay any anxieties the client may have about privacy and confidentiality of sensitive health information. When the first call is placed, after briefly introducing yourself and the name of the program, immediately ask if the communication was received and if the client has any questions. Reassure the client about privacy of information and unless the client expresses a desire to be removed from the program, proceed into the assessment.

Component	Question
General	When were you first told about the problem? ● How many years ago? ● Did you have a specific blood test or was it for another reason such as preparing for surgery or giving blood?
	How are you feeling right now?
	Are you having any new symptoms? If having new symptoms: ● When did these begin? ● Are the symptoms getting better or worse? ● What have you done about the symptoms?
	When did you see your doctor/health care provider about the symptoms? ● What did the doctor/health care provider tell you is causing the symptoms?
Medications	What medicine are you taking at this time? ● The name of the medicine? ● The dosage? ● The frequency the medicine is taken? ● If the medication needs to be taken with: ▪ Food? ▪ Fluids? ▪ Empty stomach? ▪ With another medication?

(continued)

(continued)

Component	Question
	Have you been taking the medication as prescribed? If not, • How often are you taking the medication? • What is the reason that you are skipping/missing doses? • Have you noticed a change in your health since you have been changing the frequency or dose of the medication?
	Have you had any adverse effects from the medication, such as: • Nausea and vomiting? • Abdominal pain? • Abdominal weight gain? • Thinning of the muscles of the arms and legs?
	What has your doctor or health care provider told you about the adverse effects?

PROMOTING MAXIMUM WELLNESS

Because there is no definite cure for HIV/AIDS, the goal of telephonic care is to prevent the development of opportunistic infections/ secondary cancers. Additional information that would be beneficial for these patients includes:

• Skin care
• Nutritional intake

Although the reason why the disease occurred is not a part of the assessment, patients should be encouraged to generally avoid high-risk behaviors and be referred to local support groups and resources for any specific questions or concerns.

KEY POINTS

• HIV is considered a chronic disease.
• Many people can experience healthy lives if treatment is started immediately when diagnosed and rigidly followed.

● Adverse effects and medication costs are the major reasons for nonadherence to the prescribed medication regimen.
● Medications will not cure the virus.
● Ceasing to follow the treatment plan is a major reason for the development of AIDS and subsequent opportunistic infections and secondary cancers.
● Telephonic care calls are not meant to replace individual counseling if requested or indicated.
● General positive health principles should be encouraged to include avoidance of high-risk behaviors.

BIBLIOGRAPHY

AIDS Info. Guidelines for the use of antiretroviral agents in HIV-1-infected adults and adolescents. Retrieved from https://aidsinfo.nih.gov/guidelines/html/1/adult-and-adolescent-arv-guidelines/11/what-to-start

AIDS.gov. Overview of HIV treatments. Retrieved from https://www.aids.gov/hiv-aids-basics/just-diagnosed-with-hiv-aids/treatment-options/overview-of-hiv-treatments/index.html

Howell, S. C. (2005). Disease management programs HIV/AIDS. Disease management colloquium, AIDS Healthcare Foundation, Philadelphia, PA. Retrieved from http://www.ehcca.com/presentations/dmconference3/howell_1b.pdf

Lemone, P. (2015). *Medical-surgical nursing* (6th ed.). Upper Saddle River, NJ: Pearson.

Pearson Education. (2015). *Nursing: A concept-based approach to learning* (2nd ed., Vol. 2). Upper Saddle River, NJ: Author.

Wilson, B. A., Shannon, M. T., & Shields, K. M. (2015). *Pearson nurse's drug guide 2016*. Upper Saddle River, NJ: Pearson.

Additional Aspects of Telephonic Patient/Client Care

The nurse providing telephonic care does more than call a patient/client, ask assessment questions, plan the next call, and hang up. Assessment is just the first step when using this approach for client care. But once the assessment is completed, what happens next?

Depending on the organization, health insurance plan, or disease management program, the next steps are often outlined for the nurse. For some programs this means that the client is assessed for health risk behaviors, such as smoking, alcohol intake, substance use, and inactivity. Once these behaviors are identified, protocols might be used to guide the client into changing the behaviors.

Disease management programs often have well-developed robust teaching tools that are to be used when discussing health issues with the client. However, because a disease management program for every potential illness or condition has yet to be developed, you, the nurse, must be prepared to guide and instruct the client to perform actions to minimize long-term problems and maximize health status.

Keep in mind that an infinite number of strategies and approaches can be used when conducting telephonic nursing care. There is no one "right" way to encourage someone to do something or a "wrong" way to talk about a health problem. Access your inner creativity and approach each call with an open mind. Remember, this is not a research study with rigid rules and expectations. Oftentimes, the best approaches are discovered by simple trial and error.

CHAPTER 21

Patient/Client Care

Upon completion of this chapter, the nurse will:

1. Discuss approaches when performing telephonic nursing care
2. Strategize ways to enhance patient/client learning
3. Incorporate methods to enhance patient/client acceptance and desire to maximize personal health status

TWEAKING THE NURSING PROCESS

Every nurse can recite the steps of the nursing process and most likely implements these steps without missing a beat. However, all of the steps of the nursing process are not represented in telephonic nursing care.

Assessment has been the major portion of the text so it goes without saying the importance of this step when providing telephonic care. However, clustering data and identifying appropriate nursing diagnoses are often not a part of this process. The planning of care is often standardized especially if the patient/client is in a disease management program.

That leaves implementation and evaluation. The bulk of your care will be on implementing interventions in order to help the client change behaviors. And then you will evaluate the success of the behavior change by measuring the client's outcomes through laboratory data, improvement in symptoms, adherence to medication regimens, and not being hospitalized for a complication or new health problem. Interventions in telephonic care are provided verbally and occur through teaching.

TEACHING

Telephonic teaching is a bit different than providing teaching to a client who is in the same room. Remember:

- You will not be able to see the client or the environment.
- You will not be able to see nonverbal responses or facial expressions.
- You will not be able to watch the client read a handout.
- You will not be able to see a return demonstration.

Before beginning any teaching, you need to assess what the client already knows about a particular health problem or situation. This can be accomplished by asking "can you tell me what you know about your (disease process/medication/health problem)?" Depending on the response, you can respond accordingly.

The extent of teaching and content provided will depend on the organization, health insurance plan, or wellness program. An organization may have teaching materials or guide sheets already created to be used for specific topics. But in case standardized teaching materials do not exist, the following topics and materials would be helpful to have on hand:

Topic	Teaching Material
Wellness/Health Promotion	
Smoking cessation	• Preparing to stop smoking • Advantages of smoking cessation • Ways to control your weight when quitting smoking • What to do when the urge to smoke hits • Beginning your new life as a nonsmoker
Weight management	• Calculating your body mass index • Planning for a realistic weight loss • Fad diets: why they don't work • Exercise to aid in weight loss • When to measure body weight
Exercise/ activity	• Achieving 30 minutes a day of activity • How much exercise do you really need? • Household activities as exercise • Walking versus running

(continued)

(continued)

Topic	Teaching Material
	<ul><li>Weight training for the beginner</li><li>What do "popping" sounds really mean?</li><li>Protecting the back: improve core muscles</li></ul>
Nutrition	<ul><li>Using MyPlate™</li><li>The importance of fresh fruits and vegetables</li><li>When dairy doesn't agree with you</li><li>Protein sources for the vegan</li><li>How much water do I really need to drink?</li><li>What's better: three meals a day or six smaller meals a day?</li></ul>
Disease prevention	<ul><li>Advantages of the annual influenza vaccination</li><li>Why do I need the herpes zoster vaccination at age 60?</li><li>Does the pneumonia vaccination really prevent pneumonia?</li><li>How do I know if I have high blood pressure?</li><li>How do I know if I have diabetes?</li><li>When should I see my doctor?</li><li>When should I have a colonoscopy?</li><li>When should I have a mammogram?</li><li>When should I have a prostate exam?</li><li>Why should I examine my own breasts?</li><li>How do I examine my own breasts?</li><li>Why should I examine my own testicles?</li><li>How do I examine my own testicles?</li></ul>
Rest/sleep	<ul><li>Is it insomnia or something else?</li><li>How much sleep do I really need?</li><li>Is napping important for older people?</li><li>What does loud snoring really mean?</li><li>Alcohol versus a sleeping pill: which one is better?</li></ul>
Alcohol intake	<ul><li>Maximum daily alcohol intake for men and women</li><li>Can I have alcohol with my prescribed medications?</li></ul>
Specific Health Problems	
Hypertension	<ul><li>What is a normal blood pressure?</li><li>How often should blood pressure be checked?</li><li>What can be done to lower blood pressure?</li></ul>

(continued)

(*continued*)

Topic	Teaching Material
Osteoporosis	• What causes osteoporosis? • What can be done to help osteoporosis? • What medication is used to help osteoporosis?
Arthritis	• What causes osteoarthritis? • What is the difference between osteoarthritis and rheumatoid arthritis? • What can be done to help arthritis? • How do I know if I have arthritis? • What is total joint replacement surgery?
Chest pain	• When should I worry about chest pain? • Why do I get chest pain after eating? • Why do I get chest pain when I exercise? • What is a heart attack?
Back pain	• What causes back pain? • What can be done for back pain? • Is bed rest the best treatment for back pain? • Back pain: why exercise helps

Depending on the client population, additional topics and titles can be added at any time. Some organizations have contracts with patient teaching material companies who provide complete libraries of topics online for the staff to use when appropriate. An advantage of using prepared client teaching materials is not having to pay staff to research and write the materials. A major disadvantage is that the materials may not be appropriate for the client population or may lack specific disease processes or topics.

PATIENT/CLIENT REQUESTS INFORMATION

In an ideal world, all patients/clients will want to learn everything about every diagnosed health problem and will follow teaching materials to improve health or prevent future problems. Know that this will never exist, but at times you will have a client who asks for specific information for a health problem, medication, or treatment. The client who requests information is one who is prepared to learn.

When this occurs, you will not need to assess for readiness to absorb new information or ask in-depth questions. The greatest challenge might be locating the appropriate material, if the request is not routinely asked by other clients, or spending time preparing a response.

However, prior to diving in and answering the client's question or providing teaching material, a few minor questions would be beneficial. Unfortunately, some clients may be "shopping" for information or seeking a response to a question that they "like." For example, a client may be informed about a health problem and given a specific action or actions to take to prevent the onset of disease. The client does not want to take the recommended action and asks you what should be done about the problem. Without knowing what action was already recommended, you could fall right into a trap: "My doctor told me to do this but you are telling me to do that." Protect yourself from these no-win situations and always ask first:

- What do you know about the problem?
- What did your doctor tell you to do?

The client's responses will help guide your teaching.

PATIENT/CLIENT WOULD BENEFIT FROM TEACHING MATERIAL

No one really likes to make lifestyle changes, but these can make the most impact in the shortest amount of time on a person's health status. Oftentimes, these changes are categorized as modifiable risk factors and include:

- Weight management/reduction
- Smoking cessation
- Alcohol consumption
- Substance use/abuse
- Activity/exercise
- Cholesterol/lipid levels

Each of these risk factors requires a change in behavior. Changing behavior is not easy to do, and you will need to spend some time going through the process with the client. When it is identified that a client would benefit from teaching material to alter a modifiable risk factor, several actions should occur. First, assess the client's willingness to change the behavior. A person with chronic obstructive pulmonary disease would benefit from smoking cessation; however, they have smoked 2 ppd of cigarettes for 45 years. Without a doubt, the patient/client realizes that cigarette smoking contributed (caused) the health problem; however, unless the patient/client is ready to stop smoking, talking about smoking cessation will be a waste of your time.

Instead of explaining how much better the patient/client will breathe when no longer smoking or how much money they will save by not buying cigarettes every day, begin the conversation using a nonthreatening approach such as, "Have you ever considered not smoking?" or "Have you ever tried to quit smoking?" If the patient/client is wearing oxygen at home, you might need to interject home oxygen safety information such as "remember that there should not be any smoking around oxygen because it could cause a fire." This approach does not accuse the client of doing something potentially dangerous but does adequately inform the client of the home safety risk.

A change in behavior will not occur immediately or after a few brief telephone calls. It may take weeks or months before a client will even consider making a change. Avoid starting each conversation about the behavior that needs to be changed because the client may start avoiding the telephone calls. The behavior change issue should be gently approached such as "since our last call have you thought any more about quitting smoking?" Although this is a closed-ended question, the client will most likely respond with ether a "yes" or "no" and then proceed to defend the answer. Remain aloof when hearing the client's response and gently reinforce any information or teaching that was provided on the previous call. Unless the client is ready to make a change, going forward with additional teaching material will be futile.

PATIENT/CLIENT IS READY TO MAKE A CHANGE

The first indication that a change in behavior is on the horizon is when the patient/client says something like "I saw on television some medicine to help stop smoking," or "my cousin quit smoking and he only gained 5 lb." The client brings up the subject, makes a comment, or asks a question. The door may only be slightly cracked open, but this is probably the only invitation you will receive, so walk right in.

The change process has been reviewed numerous times throughout nursing school; however, a brief review might be beneficial. Depending on the resource used, the change process can have anywhere from three to six stages.

The Lewin Model

One of the simplest models for change, the Lewin model, has three phases:

- Unfreeze
- Make the change
- Refreeze

Unfreeze

Unfreezing occurs when it is identified that a change needs to be made and steps are taken to release previously held beliefs, behaviors, or patterns. For someone who is thinking about smoking cessation, this could mean investigating nicotine replacement products, discussing smoking cessation medication with the health care provider, or researching smoking cessation materials on the Internet.

Make the change

In this phase, the action occurs. So for the person desiring to stop smoking, a day is planned when smoking will no longer occur.

Refreeze

This last phase is probably the most difficult because the new changed behavior is to be practiced. Unless the person has support, refreezing the new behavior may not occur. An example of this might be someone who has repeatedly attempted to quit smoking but has not been successful. The new behavior is not freezing.

The Transtheoretical Model of Change

Developed by Prochaska and DiClemente in 1983, this model is one of the most widely used in nursing practice. According to this model, there are five phases to the change process:

- Precontemplation
- Contemplation

- Preparation
- Action
- Maintenance

Precontemplation

In this phase, the person is not ready to make any behavior changes. If asked about a certain behavior, the person may respond with "don't talk to me about that" or "I'm not going to do it so don't even bother discussing it."

Contemplation

In this stage, the person is "thinking about" changing a behavior. The person may research the change being considered, ask questions, and consider how the change will affect the person's life.

Preparation

In the preparation stage, the person has decided to make the change. At this time, the person may experiment with the change periodically, just to see how it "feels" or if it "can be done."

Action

When this stage has been reached, the change has occurred. The biggest issue during this stage is the risk for relapse. The behavior being practiced is still very new and resorting to a previous practice or behavior can occur at any time.

Maintenance

Those in the maintenance phase have been using the new behavior for a longer period of time. The threat (or fear) of relapse is still present although at less intensity than during the action phase.

APPLICATION OF CHANGE THEORY TO TELEPHONIC NURSING CARE

The following is an example of a series of conversations that could occur as a client works through the phases of change during telephonic nursing care calls. In this scenario, a middle-aged patient/client in the diabetes disease management program has been directed by the health care provider to lose 50 lb.

Nurse	Patient/Client
Precontemplation	
I see here that you were scheduled for a doctor's appointment last week. How did that go?	Oh, I went to the doctor alright. He told me to lose 50 lb or plan my funeral. It was my choice.
Oh my, how do you feel about that?	Don't you think that if I could lose weight that I would have by now? I see all of those TV commercials for weight loss plans and clubs and I'm just not interested. Let's talk about something else . . .
Contemplation	
It's been 2 weeks since we last talked. How have your blood sugars been running?	They could be better. You know, I was thinking that if I did drop a few pounds, I might not need to check my blood sugars that often. That would save me some money on those strips. And, I could cut back on my grocery bills too.
It sounds like you are thinking about changing your diet.	Yes, that's it though. I'm thinking about it. It won't be easy. I meet my buddies at the bar a couple of times a week for pizza and beer and what would they say if I said, light beer for me and a salad. That would get a good laugh.
What makes you think they would laugh?	I just know those guys. Anybody who changes anything is ribbed for weeks. Although when I think about it, they could stand to lose a few pounds too!
Preparation	
How was your vacation?	Terrific but there was way too much food on that cruise and I ended up gaining more weight. I'm glad I went, though, because that was my last splurge before I start my diet.
So you've decided to start a diet?	Yes, that's right. I'm starting on Monday of next week. I'm giving myself a few more days to throw out food that isn't good for me and surround myself with only the good stuff.

(continued)

(*continued*)

Nurse	Patient/Client
What type of diet are you planning to follow?	Well, I went on a website and read through a lot of the popular ones like high protein and no carbohydrate, but those wouldn't work for me with diabetes. So I called my doctor and talked with the dietician there, and she suggested that I follow an 1,800-calorie eating plan. She sent me a few papers explaining the kinds of food that I should eat instead of the garbage that I've been eating for years. It's going to take time to get used to this but I think I'm ready to do this now.
Action	
It's been several weeks since we last talked. I see here that you had to go out of town for work a few weeks ago. How have you been doing?	Yeah, I had to go to Illinois for a business meeting and ended up staying for a week for a special project. It was ok. I had started my diet 2 weeks before I left so I had dropped a few pounds and felt better in my suits. I was staying in a really nice hotel that had room service, and they had heart-healthy meals listed. I was able to stick to my diet and have lost a total of 7 lb so far.
Wow! Good for you! You must be really happy with the results so far.	I am. Now I'm really motivated to lose this weight. My doctor is going to pass out the next time he weighs me for an appointment. But even better, my blood sugars are around 90 every morning. That's a huge improvement for me!
Action (relapse)	
How've you been doing? We talked 2 weeks ago and you were going to visit your brother in South Carolina.	I'm much better now. I did go to see my brother and his family, and his wife is a good cook—too good! I cheated every day I was visiting with them. She makes the best fried chicken and my twin nephews had a birthday so there was homemade birthday cake and the best ice cream I've ever had. I gained 4 lb in 1 week.

(*continued*)

(*continued*)

Nurse	Patient/Client
What have you done since returning from your trip?	Oh I started right back up again. I actually cut my calories down a few hundred for several days just to try to get this bloat off of me.
It's not easy making changes to an eating plan. Slipping up is part of the process.	You don't have to tell me! I know that for sure. But I'm ok and still committed to losing this weight. My next doctor's appointment is in 4 months. I might not lose the entire 50 lb by then but I will have a good amount off.
Maintenance	
I see here that you've been following an 1,800 calorie eating plan now for 3 months. How's it been going for you?	Great! Well, it would be better if I didn't have to be eating this way but it's going great.
How much weight have you lost so far?	27 lb and my doctor's appointment is in 2 weeks. I want to lose 3 more lb. so that I will have lost 30 lb since my last appointment.
How have your blood sugars been since you've lost the weight?	They haven't been above 90 for weeks now. I only check it in the morning now, which has been great.
Are you still meeting up with your friends at the bar?	Oh we still meet but get this, my one buddy's wife started hounding him to lose weight so he asked me about my diet. I showed it to him and he asked me if the other guys would mind meeting at a different place to watch the games. So last week, we met at a different sports bar that had a better menu and we both got light beer. The guys didn't say a word.
I am so happy for your success. Is there anything that I can send you to help keep you on track?	Well, I think I need to get some kind of exercise. I walk the dog every night after work, but I don't think that's enough. Do you have anything about activity or exercise that you can send me? I can take it with me to my doctor's appointment and let him look at it too.

Hopefully, this example gives you some idea of the type of conversation/dialogue you might experience when assisting a client work through the stages of change. Keep in mind that progression through the stages will not always go as planned. A patient/client may be contemplating a change one week and then 2 weeks later resort back to precontemplation. During the next call, the client may be discussing preparation and then get cold feet. A few months later, the client may be in contemplation but still have misgivings about making the change. This process can go on for months. The best thing to do is to not get discouraged. No one can make anyone do anything that they are not prepared to do. Your role is to provide information, answer questions, and be the client's number one fan.

IDENTIFY TEACHABLE MOMENTS

In a perfect world, a client will listen to advice provided by the health care professional, discuss options for changes during care calls, plan and implement changes, and then proceed with improved health. Well, it does not work that way. Clients may not be aware of a change that can be made, and it is up to you to bring the potential change to their attention.

A phrase that has been bantered around for several years would be essential for you to remember when contacting clients over the telephone: we don't know what we don't know. In other words, it is impossible to know everything, and because we don't know everything, we don't know what we don't know. Sounds complicated but it is quite simple. A person cannot be expected to make a change if the person is unaware of what the change is supposed to do or what it means.

When engaging in telephonic care, you will be collecting assessment data and helping the client implement actions to improve health. The client with hypertension may make a statement such as "I've been taking my pills and not using salt, but my blood pressure still won't come down below 140." This could be your opportunity to talk about adding exercise to the mix to help with blood pressure control. A statement such as "how much activity do you get every day" would be a good opening to talk about exercise.

The number of teachable moments during telephonic care can be endless. Examples for these moments are as follows:

Conversation Content	Teachable Moment
Wants to have a cigarette after eating a meal	• Encourage to go to nonsmoking restaurants • Make the home a no smoking zone
Does not have time to exercise	• Take the steps instead of the elevator at work • Take a walk around the block during lunch time • Park the car farther from the front door at work • Walk to the corner mailbox instead of driving to the post office
Misses half and half in the morning coffee	Suggest almond milk in coffee
Misses having burgers for lunch	Suggest ordering a burger and eating it without the bun
Wants to go to happy hour after work on Fridays but doesn't want to drink sugary beverages	Suggest wine spritzer or light beer
Doesn't have time to eat breakfast in the morning	• Suggest making hard boiled eggs and have them in the refrigerator • Suggest adding protein powder to morning coffee
Orders out for lunch every day	• Suggest packing a lunch from leftovers from the previous evening's dinner meal • Suggest eating half of the lunch and saving it for the next day or having it later for dinner
Wants to have a cigarette with morning coffee	Suggest changing morning beverage to tea
Can't remember to take morning pills before leaving for work	Place the medication in the bathroom next to the toothbrush

(continued)

(continued)

Conversation Content	Teachable Moment

Doesn't like to exercise	● Suggest approaching household chores as activity
	  ▪ Walk around the bed several times while making it
	  ▪ Pick up clothing from the floor one item at a time
	  ▪ Use broad strokes when wiping down kitchen counters
	  ▪ Do leg raises or walk in place while washing the dishes, folding clothes
	● Perform leg stretches while putting on socks in the morning
	● Stand when talking on the telephone
	● Get up and walk during a commercial when watching television in the evening

Skips breakfast and lunch and is ravenous by dinner time	● Place healthy snacks in desk at work:
	  ▪ Almonds
	  ▪ Pumpkin seeds
	● Drink a glass of water before eating
	● Start the evening meal with a small bowl of bouillon or broth soup

Craves salty snacks	● Make air popped popcorn in the microwave and use 1/3 less sodium salt
Craves sweet snacks	● Make sugar-free gelatin and low-fat whipped topping ● Substitute apple sauce for sugar and oil when baking ● Make boxed cake mixes with one 12 ounce can of diet soda instead of adding butter, eggs, and milk (for yellow/white cake mix use one 12 ounce can diet ginger ale; for chocolate cake mix use one 12 ounce can diet cola)

(continued)

(continued)

Conversation Content	Teachable Moment
Craves cigarettes when watching television	• Suggest keeping hands busy with needlework (knitting, crocheting) • Suggest getting up and rearranging a kitchen shelf or other activity while still being able to hear the television
Wants to walk but does not live in an area that is safe (no sidewalks), or inclement weather conditions, or needs assistance with a walker or canes	• Suggest going to a shopping area or mall to walk • Suggest walking in a grocery store and using the shopping cart as support

Remember that these are just suggestions and you might think of others that are just as effective. The intention is to support the client to perform actions that will either change an undesirable behavior or reinforce a desirable behavior.

KEEPING THE LINES OF COMMUNICATION OPEN

The nurse providing telephonic care is just one member of the patient's/client's health care team. The client will be making routine health care provider appointments, having laboratory or diagnostic testing, recovering from surgery, or participating in rehabilitative sessions. You will be contacting the client in addition to, and not in place of, these other health care–related activities.

Because of this, a client might not understand the purpose of your calls. A client may say "I see my doctor and several specialists who provide my care, and I don't need to talk to you, too." Although this might seem a valid argument, at times seeing physicians is not enough. As the telephonic nurse, you will be:

- Reinforcing the medical treatment plan
- Encouraging positive changes
- Assessing for changes in health status
- Answering questions about disease processes
- Recommending approaches for medication compliance
- Being someone to talk to when the health status becomes overwhelming

Always encourage the client to discuss the content of the care calls with their health care provider. Telephonic nurses rarely contact health care providers so the client must be empowered to share information learned during care calls during the next office appointment. Some clients have asked the health care provider to write down the results of laboratory and diagnostic tests so they can be shared during the next telephonic care call. As electronic medical records are becoming more commonplace in health care provider offices, receiving copies of laboratory data and testing reports should not be an issue.

If asked about starting something that the client has never done before, such as an exercise program or other activity, gently remind the client to discuss the exercise plan with their health care provider before beginning the activity. It is possible that a client has a health problem that is not well documented or the patient/client is not explaining very well. An activity may be contraindicated for the client based on a health problem.

Remember not to take any derogatory client statements to heart. The client just may not know the purpose of the calls or the overall goal and intention. Take the time to explain this information. Realize though that some clients may think you are trying to sell them something and will hang up. Because of this, some telephonic nurses have adopted a conversation opening such as "Hello, my name is Linda and I'm calling from your health plan. This is not a sales call." And if that does not work and the client still does not want to take your calls, consider disenrolling them from the program.

KEY POINTS

- The nursing process is modified when providing telephonic nursing care.
- The major intervention in telephonic nursing care is teaching.
- Having a "stash" of patient teaching material available during care calls is invaluable.
- Change can be a painful process. There are several stages to this process, which do not always proceed in an orderly manner.
- Take the patient's/client's lead when discussing a change in behavior. Provide information and support along the way. Never take a patient's/client's resistance to change personally.

- Take the time during care calls to capitalize on teachable moments. If a patient/client asks a question about something that means they are interested in learning more about the situation, do your best. If you don't know the answer to something, immediately tell the patient/client that you will call back with the information as soon as it is available.
- Keep in mind the purpose of the care calls. Always encourage patients/clients to discuss the calls with the health care provider and reinforce discussing any changes in activity or exercise with the health care provider before beginning the activity or exercise.
- Do not take it personally if patients/clients do not want to participate in a telephonic program. They may change their mind in the days or weeks ahead and call you back.

BIBLIOGRAPHY

Kent, R. H. (2011). Unfreeze/refreeze: A simple change model. *The Mansis Development Corporation*. Retrieved from http://www.mansis.com/wp-content/uploads/2013/01/A-Simple-Change-Model1.pdf

Lickerman, A. (2009). 5 steps to changing any behavior. *Psychology Today*. Retrieved from https://www.psychologytoday.com/blog/happiness-in-world/200910/5-steps-changing-any-behavior

Nursing Theories. (2016). Stages of change model/transtheoretical model (TTM). Retrieved from http://currentnursing.com/nursing_theory/transtheoretical_model.html

Pro-Change Behavior Systems. (2016). The transtheoretical model. Retrieved from http://www.prochange.com/transtheoretical-model-of-behavior-change

Prochaska, J. O., & DiClemente, C. C. (1984). *The transtheoretical approach: Towards a systematic eclectic framework*. Homewood, IL: Dow Jones-Irwin.

CHAPTER 22

Review of Laboratory Values and Diagnostic Tests

LEARNING OUTCOMES

Upon completion of this chapter, the nurse will:

1. Summarize the types of diagnostic and laboratory tests appropriate for reporting through telephonic care
2. Analyze ways to discuss the importance of diagnostic and laboratory tests with clients
3. Strategize approaches to enhance client adherence to diagnostic and laboratory testing regimens

IMPORTANCE OF LABORATORY AND DIAGNOSTIC TESTS

Diagnostic and laboratory testing is an integral part of telephonic nursing care. These tests are used to:

- Identify participation in disease management programs
- Evaluate compliance with the prescribed treatment plan
- Analyze the impact of teaching interventions on client health status

This chapter is not to replace any diagnostic and laboratory textbooks but rather is intended to highlight diagnostic and laboratory tests that you might most frequently encounter when providing telephonic care.

TYPES OF DIAGNOSTIC TESTS

Generally, a client in a wellness program will not be scheduled or reporting the results of diagnostic testing unless a symptom or problem occurs. The types of tests prescribed for the client will be closely associated with a suspected disease process and used to either rule out a problem or confirm the diagnosis. The following table categorizes the types of diagnostic tests that you might need to explain when conducting telephonic care. Keep in mind when explaining a diagnostic test that the most basic language and terms should be used. The associated teaching column in the table provides suggestions to use when explaining the test.

Health Problem	Diagnostic Test	Associated Teaching
Integumentary disorders	Biopsy	Takes a piece of the skin and tests it for infections
Respiratory disorders	Pulmonary function tests	Checks to see how much obstruction or constriction is in the lungs
	Bronchoscopy	Examines the lungs and breathing airway to check for obstructions/tumors or bleeding
	Chest x-ray	Looks at the major structures in the chest in relation to the location of the lungs
Cardiovascular disorders	EKG	Examines the electrical activity of the heart
	Echocardiogram	• Checks the valves in the heart • Indirectly measures the functioning of the left ventricle in the form of ejection fraction
	Cardiac catheterization	Checks the arteries and other structures in the heart
	Venogram/Doppler studies	Uses sound waves to check for any blood clots in the blood vessel
	Stress/treadmill test	Determines the function of the heart during exercise
Gastrointestinal (GI) disorders	Abdominal x-ray	Checks for any blockages or if there is free air in the bowel

(continued)

(continued)

Health Problem	Diagnostic Test	Associated Teaching
	Abdominal ultrasound	Checks the structures in the abdomen to include the pancreas, liver, and gallbladder for any blockages, stones, or masses
	Endoscopy	Looks at the esophagus and the lining of the stomach to check for ulcers or tumors
	Colonoscopy	Looks at the lining and structure of the colon to check for polyps, ulcers, or tumors
	Upper GI/barium swallow	By drinking barium, the lining of the stomach and small intestine are examined for ulcers or blockages
	Lower GI/barium enema	By using barium through an enema, the lining of the large intestine is examined for ulcers or blockages
	Liver biopsy	Takes a small piece of the liver to check it for any problems with function
Musculoskeletal disorders	X-rays	Looks for any breaks in the bones
	CT scan/MRI	Looks for any problems within the bones like a mass/tumor
	Arthroscopy	Looks at the structures associated with a joint for any breaks or tears in the tissue around the joint
Neurologic disorders	Electromyogram/ nerve conduction studies (EMGS/ NCVs)	Checks the electrical activity generated by the nerves that feed the muscles
	Myelogram	• Looks at the nerves that originate from the spinal cord • Checks for blood flow to the nerve and for any compression from the bones in the back (vertebrae)

(continued)

(*continued*)

Health Problem	Diagnostic Test	Associated Teaching
	CT scan/MRI	Looks at the brain and spinal cord for any problems with blood flow, broken skull bones, broken spinal bones, and if there are any masses/tumors or bleeding
Sensory disorders	Tonometry	Checks for the amount of pressure within the eyes
	Audiometry	Tests for hearing
Genitourinary disorders	CT scan of the kidneys	Checks for any problems with blood flow to the kidneys or if there are any masses/tumors/kidney stones
	Cystoscopy	Looks directly at the bladder to check for any irritation or masses/tumors
	Intravenous pyelogram	Injects dye to look at the kidneys and check for stones
	Renal biopsy	Takes a piece of the kidney to check for a specific disease
	Prostate biopsy	Takes a piece of the prostate to check for diseases
	Prostate ultrasound	Checks to see the size of the prostate and if the enlargement is pressing on any other body tissues
	Breast biopsy	Takes a piece of the breast tissue to check if a swelling/mass is cancerous
	Breast ultrasound	Uses sound waves to look at a breast mass to see if it is solid or filled with fluid (cyst)
	Laparoscopy	Looks at the organs in the (female) abdomen to check for location, swellings/masses, or blockages
	Mammogram	Looks at the structures within the breasts to check for masses/tumors

TYPES OF LABORATORY TESTS

The volume of laboratory tests that could be prescribed and reported on by the client receiving telephonic care can be quite lengthy. Oftentimes, the client is unaware of what is being tested and will ask you why something was being done. The following table provides a general list of laboratory tests that may be prescribed for the clients receiving telephonic care.

Health Problem	Sample Source	Laboratory Test	Associated Teaching
Integumentary disorders	Scraping	Culture	Small pieces of skin taken to see if an infection is caused by bacteria, virus, or fungus
Respiratory disorders	Sputum	Culture	Sputum/phlegm is examined for bacteria causing an infection
	Sputum	Cytology	Sputum/phlegm is examined for cancer cells
	Blood	Complete blood count	Blood sample to check if the number of white blood cells that fight infection are increased
Cardiovascular disorders	Blood	Lipid panel	• Blood sample to check for the amount of the different kinds of fat in the blood ▪ Triglycerides: fatty acids in the blood ▪ Cholesterol types: – LDL: low-density lipoproteins; considered the "bad" cholesterol; helps determine the effects of diabetes and contributes to heart disease

(continued)

(*continued*)

Health Problem	Sample Source	Laboratory Test	Associated Teaching
			– HDL: high-density lipoproteins; considered the "good" cholesterol; helps measure the effects of exercise and diet changes on body fat levels to prevent heart disease
	Blood	Complete blood count	• Blood sample to check for the number and amount of red blood cells that carry oxygen • Blood sample to check for the shape, size, and amount of different blood cells to diagnose blood diseases
	Blood	Erythrocyte sedimentation rate	Blood sample to check for inflammation that occurs in heart disease
	Blood	B-type natriuretic peptide	Blood test to check for congestive heart failure
	Blood	Troponin	Blood test that measures damage to the heart muscle after a heart attack
	Blood	Prothrombin time/ International Normalized Ratio (INR)	• Blood test to measure how long it takes for blood to clot • Used to adjust blood thinner (warfarin) medication
GI disorders	Stool	Guaiac	• Used to see if there is blood in the stool • Checks for bleeding in the stomach and intestines
	Blood	Serum amylase	Checks to see if pancreas inflammation is improving

(*continued*)

(continued)

Health Problem	Sample Source	Laboratory Test	Associated Teaching
	Blood	Liver function	Checks all of the different enzymes that can be altered by medication, infections like hepatitis, or cirrhosis
	Blood	Glucose	• Used to measure the amount of sugar in the blood • Helps determine pancreas function and if treatment for diabetes is being effective
	Blood	Albumin	Measures the amount of protein in the blood
Musculoskeletal disorders	Blood	Calcium	• Checks to see how much calcium is in the blood and the bones • Helps determine if bones are strong or brittle
	Blood	Vitamin D	Measures the amount of this vitamin in the blood because it helps with bone development and strength
	Blood	Uric acid	• Uric acid is made by the body by the metabolism of certain kinds of foods • Increases in this level can cause gout • Checking this level helps determine if treatment for gout is effective
	Blood	Rheumatoid factor	Checks to see if arthritis is being caused by wear and tear or inflammation in the body
Neurologic disorders	Spinal fluid	Lumbar puncture	Checks to see if a health problem is being caused by an infection

(continued)

(continued)

Health Problem	Sample Source	Laboratory Test	Associated Teaching
Genitourinary disorders	Blood	Blood urea nitrogen	• Checks to see if the body is eliminating wastes through the urine • Measures the effectiveness of dialysis
	Blood	Creatinine	• Checks to see if the body is eliminating wastes through the urine • Measures the effectiveness of dialysis
	Blood	Potassium	• Checks to see the amount of potassium in the body, which can be altered in kidney diseases • Measures the effectiveness of dialysis
	Blood	Phosphorus	• Checks to see the amount of phosphorus in the body, which can be altered in kidney diseases • Measures if the diet or dialysis needs to be changed
	Urine	Urinalysis	Measures the different types of wastes that are removed from the body through the urine
	Urine	Culture	Checks to see if there is an infection in the urine causing a health problem
	Urine	Albumin	• Measures the amount of protein that is in the urine • Used to determine kidney function that can be altered because of kidney disease or diabetes

(continued)

(continued)

Health Problem	Sample Source	Laboratory Test	Associated Teaching
	Blood	Prostate-specific antigen	Measures the amount of a substance produced by the prostate to determine if the prostate is functioning well or stressed by cancer
	Blood	Venereal disease research lab (VDRL)	Checks for syphilis, a sexually transmitted infection
	Blood	Testosterone	• Measures the amount of this hormone in the blood • Used to help diagnose infertility • Used to help identify sexual characteristic changes
	Vagina	Chlamydia	Checks for chlamydia, a sexually transmitted infection
	Vagina	Culture	Checks for infections caused by bacteria or yeast
	Vagina	Pap	• Checks for cancer cells in the vagina and cervix • Sometimes used to measure effectiveness of hormone replacement therapy
	Vagina	Human papilloma virus (HPV)	• Done with a Pap test • Checks to see if an HPV infection is present
	Blood	Estrogen	• Measures the amount of this hormone in the blood • Used to help diagnose the status of menopause

(continued)

(continued)

Health Problem	Sample Source	Laboratory Test	Associated Teaching
HIV/AIDS	Blood	CD4 (T-lymphocyte)	• Measures the effectiveness of medications used for the treatment of HIV • Checks for the onset of AIDS
Diabetes	Blood	Hemoglobin A1c	• Checked every 3 months • Measures control of blood sugar levels over the previous 3 months

CLIENT ADHERENCE

No one likes to have blood drawn or have to place a small amount of body fluid into a cup. Scheduling for diagnostic tests can be a nightmare if work schedules need to be changed or there are issues with child care. But, ongoing diagnostic or laboratory testing is essential when evaluating the effectiveness of telephonic care.

Yes, having to collect specimens or arrive to an outpatient facility for testing is an inconvenience to the client, but the alternative could be hospitalization or surgery. Clients need to be encouraged to keep scheduled appointments for blood work, especially if medication dose adjustments will be made.

One of your many roles when contacting the clients is to:

• Remind them to schedule a blood test
• Keep an appointment for a blood test
• Schedule a follow-up appointment with the health care provider to receive blood test results

You can adjust the content of your conversation accordingly. For example, an initial call might be "don't forget to call and schedule an appointment for your hemoglobin A1c." Then in 2 weeks you can ask "did you make your appointment for the hemoglobin A1c?" If so, then the follow-up call might be, "did you get your hemoglobin A1c results yet?" This approach can be used for any of the diagnostic/laboratory tests that the client is to routinely have completed.

INTERPRETING RESULTS

At times, a client may want to hear what you have to say about the results of a laboratory or diagnostic test. There are many reasons why someone asks for "another opinion" but keep in mind the scope of nursing practice and always refer the client to discuss the results with the health care provider. You cannot go wrong by asking in response "what did your doctor say to you about the test?" This way you will know what the client has been informed about the findings. From there you can talk about the proposed treatment such as changes in medication, activity, diet, or surgery.

KEY POINTS

- Ongoing diagnostic and laboratory tests are an integral part of telephonic care.
- Diagnostic and laboratory tests are used to identify participation in disease management programs, evaluate client compliance with the prescribed treatment plan, and determine effectiveness of teaching interventions provided.
- Although there is a myriad of diagnostic and laboratory tests available, not all are appropriate or necessary for the client receiving telephonic care.
- Remind clients when diagnostic/laboratory tests are due and routinely follow up to encourage adherence. The results help determine if your interventions have been effective.
- Keep in mind your scope of nursing practice. Always refer the client back to the health care provider for clarification on a finding from a diagnostic or laboratory test.

BIBLIOGRAPHY

Lemone, P. (2015). *Medical-surgical nursing* (6th ed.). Upper Saddle River, NJ: Pearson.

Pearson Education. (2015). *Nursing: A concept-based approach to learning* (2nd ed., Vol. 2). Upper Saddle River, NJ: Author.

Van Leeuwen, A. M., & Bladh, M. L. (2015). *Comprehensive handbook of laboratory & diagnostic tests* (6th ed.). Philadelphia, PA: F. A. Davis.

CHAPTER 23

Documentation

Upon completion of this chapter, the nurse will:

1. Examine the types of information that should be documented for telephonic care
2. Master the clinical documentation system used by the organization/ health plan/wellness program
3. Achieve a comfort level documenting while conducting a telephone conversation

INFORMATION

Without a doubt, you will be collecting a large amount of information, but you will need to know where to place this information within your clinical information system. Documentation would be so much easier if every organization, health plan, or wellness program used the same computer software for documentation, but this is not the case.

The first thing you will have to do is learn the computer software system. The most common platform for these software programs is a Windows-based operating system or something that closely resembles Windows. What this means is there are individual windows or screens that open up when a link is accessed. In layman's terms, this means that when a word is in a different color, clicking the word will cause another screen or window to open up. Sometimes, the word that is to be clicked may also be underlined or *italicized*.

Some software applications may have a list of file folders along the left column of the screen. Each folder has a different part of the medical record. When the folder is clicked, the contents appear on the main screen.

The contents of a medical record for a client receiving telephonic care would include headings such as:

- Demographics
- Past health history
- Current health problems
- Physical assessment data
- Medications
- Diagnostic tests
- Laboratory tests
- Health plan information/wellness program information
- Mailings/materials
- Health plan/disease management claims data

Keep in mind that this list is in no particular order. Your organization or program might have them listed or categorized in a different way.

Demographics

This is usually a good place to start when contacting a client. Demographics includes:

- Name
- Address
- Telephone number(s)
- Best day and time to call
- E-mail address
- Next of kin/family member

The content is entered into a "field" or a blank space to type information. Depending on the health plan, disease management, or wellness program, most of this information may already be populated, or filled in. You will need to validate this information for accuracy. Be sure to collect all possible telephone numbers for the client. If the client is providing you with a hardline work address, ask if you have permission to contact the client at work to discuss the client's health. Employers differ in their policies about personal telephone calls during work hours.

With the use of social media, many clients may have Facebook pages and Instagram and Twitter accounts. If your software application has fields for this information in demographics, ask the client for this information as well. Keep in mind that communicating personal health information is not appropriate through Facebook, Instagram, or Twitter.

E-mail is becoming a preferred route to receive information. This may be used to remind the client of an upcoming scheduled care call or to send a client requested information about a teaching need. If the e-mail account is to a work address, check to make sure that the client is permitted to receive personal information through the account. Employers have policies about the use of e-mail for personal affairs, and depending on the policy, the employer may be able to read/access the employee's e-mails. This could be a potential violation of privacy laws.

When documenting telephone numbers, designate if it is a mobile/smartphone device or a landline. If the client only has a mobile device, when you call them, ask if they are able to talk in a secure location. It would be unacceptable to discuss the latest results of blood work or a urinalysis while a client is grocery shopping or driving children to soccer practice.

Determine the best day and time to call the client when scheduling subsequent care calls. Some clients work during the day and will only be available for evening calls. Others are unable to take calls unless they occur on Saturday morning. Most health plans and disease management/wellness programs do not make scheduled care calls on Sundays; however, Saturday calls can be commonplace.

The "next of kin" or name of a family member may or may not be in your software. Some organizations, health plans, and wellness programs ask for permission to talk with a family member about the client's health in the event that the client is hospitalized or unable to be reached for whatever reasons. This permission must be obtained from the client and documented as received by the client including the date the permission was received.

Past Health History

Again, depending on the organization, health plan, or program, this information may be prepopulated or blank. If it is prepopulated, ask the client to validate each item listed in the past health history. Keep in mind that errors can occur. A client who might have lost consciousness from heat exposure could have an entire battery of chemistry laboratory tests conducted. The health plan coders see that tests such as blood glucose were examined and automatically categorize the client as having diabetes. When the past health history information is populated in the software, diabetes appears as a past health problem. But, when you ask the client about the health problem, the client denies it exists. You will have to alter this entry so that it correctly reflects the client's previous health problems.

If the fields are not populated, you will need to spend a few minutes asking the client about previous hospitalizations and/or surgeries. For someone in a wellness program, this part of the documentation process might be completed quickly. For someone in a disease management program or someone who is older, this part may take some time to complete. Be careful, thorough, and avoid rushing through this part of documentation.

Current Health Problems

Some might say that this part of the record is obvious because the client is enrolled in a disease management program, but that is not necessarily the case. People can and do have more than one health problem, all of which are not necessarily being treated through health insurance claims. An example might be the person who has asthma and is in a disease management program for this disorder. The client also works full time and has chronic neck and low back pain. The client has not seen a physician for the pain and chooses to use chiropractic medicine; however, chiropractic care is not a part of the client's health benefits. Unless you ask about other health problems, there is no way of knowing that the client has neck and back pain.

When asking if a health problem is current, validate that the client is receiving some sort of treatment or medication for the problem now. A client may say that he or she is allergic to pet dander but has no pets, is not exposed to pets, and does not take any medication for the allergy. This health problem would most appropriately be documented as a past medical problem.

If you are assessing current health problems with an older client, take a few minutes and ask about different body areas. For example, do you have any problems with your vision or hearing? Your heart? Your breathing? Your joints or muscles? Your stomach or digestion? Being able to go to the bathroom without problems? An older client might have a chronic health problem that has existed for decades and not consider it a current health problem.

Another way to determine the existence of a current health problem is when you review current medications with the client. A person might deny having any other health problems but are prescribed a diuretic and beta blocker. These medications might be prescribed to treat hypertension, but the client considers these "pills" as something for the "blood pressure." High blood pressure is not always considered a health problem by everyone.

Physical Assessment Data

The majority of this text explains the major systems to include with physical assessment data. The software system will have categories to complete for the major areas. Ideally, the software will also have an area to add "other" information that may not be included under a major heading. Or this text might have identified a health problem in one category, and your software application has it identified somewhere else. For example, a stroke is caused by a cardiovascular problem; however, it affects the neurologic system. Some software programs might have stroke under cardiovascular system, and in others it may appear under neurologic system. Another example would be post-polio syndrome. This syndrome may be documented under either musculoskeletal or neurologic systems.

Use this text as a resource when conducting the physical assessment portion of the conversation. Remember to ask, first, if the client has any issues or problems with a major body system before diving in and asking many questions, all of which can potentially be answered as "no."

Medications

Documenting the client's current medications can be tedious but is necessary. Before embarking on this part of the documentation, ask the client to collect all of the medication vials and have them near the telephone. Then have the client read the medication bottle to you, one by one. If you do not recognize something that the client is saying, ask the client to spell the medication and to spell out the words after the name of the medication. Ask also for the date of the last refill and when the prescription needs to be renewed.

Ask the client about any known allergies to medications or foods. This information is usually documented somewhere on the medications screen by either checking a box next to no known allergies or completing a field categorized as "allergies with." If the client has no known allergies, type in the field the word "none."

You will also need to ask the client about any medications or substances the client takes that are not obtained from a prescription. This includes over-the-counter analgesics (acetaminophen/Tylenol, ibuprofen/Motrin, aspirin), expectorants (guaifenesin/Mucinex), topical agents (hydrocortisone cream), sleeping aids, and vitamin supplements/nutraceuticals/herbal remedies. Some clients do not consider over-the-counter items as medications and will not automatically include these in a list of things that the client routinely takes. Vitamin supplements/nutraceuticals/herbal remedies are rarely acknowledged as medications so you will definitely have to ask about their use. When discussing vitamin supplements/nutraceuticals/herbal remedies, ask for:

- The name of the item
- The dose
- The number of times taken each day
- The reason/expected effects
- The length of time taking the item

If the item is a blend, ask the client to read to you the list of the contents in each pill that is listed on the back of the bottle or container. Some preparations should not be taken with prescribed medications, and you might find yourself discussing how a supplement is doing more harm than good. This is also a good time to ask if the health care provider is aware of the client taking the supplement/nutraceutical/herbal preparation. Nonprescribed supplements are not controlled by the Food and Drug Administration (FDA), and the client could easily be taking something that could interfere with a medication's intended benefit or contribute to an adverse reaction.

When caring for an older client, listen carefully to the medications and be alert for possible polypharmacy. Older clients may see various health care providers, all of whom may be prescribing medications for a specific health problem. Clients may be prescribed the same medication; however, it is prescribed in a different way. For example, a client may have a prescription for furosemide from the "heart doctor" but the "kidney doctor" prescribes Lasix. The client is taking doses of each, every day. These situations need to be brought to the client's attention, thoroughly documented, and reported to the prescribing health care providers immediately.

Diagnostic Tests

This section can either be completed quickly or painstakingly filled out. It just depends on the client's memory and the name of the test. Some clients might know that an electrocardiogram is an ECG/EKG, but another client might explain a test as being one where "I had to eat nothing after midnight; I was given a shot of dye that felt warm; then I had to lay on a table for an hour while the dye went through my body." Your skills as private investigator would be most helpful at this time. You may find yourself asking what was prescribed after the test such as a new medication or surgery or asking the client if the test was done for the heart, kidneys, or brain.

Laboratory Tests

Laboratory tests can be another challenge to complete. Some older clients with diabetes may consider all blood tests to "check for sugar." You may need to ask the frequency of getting the test (every 3 months might be a hemoglobin A1c) or checking it once a week (prothrombin/INR), and then a medication dose is changed (warfarin). A client may refer to a blood test as "something to check my prostate" or to "see if there's an infection in the blood."

The best advice for you at this time is to do the best that you can obtaining the information. If the laboratory test is completed frequently, there will be claims data to help figure out what the test is and what it was used to diagnose or evaluate.

It would be ideal for every client to know the results of recent laboratory tests but not all clients will. Some clients will say that "unless the doctor calls them" they "don't worry" about the results. Other clients keep a notebook of the laboratory test, the date, and the result. It all depends on the client's willingness to keep track of the data.

Health Plan Information/Wellness Program Information

This area of the software should be populated with specific information about the program in which the client is enrolled. It might have a field that shows the date that information was mailed to the client and have a box for you to check if the client recalls receiving the information. There also might be a checkbox and a field to complete if the client decides to "opt out" or not participate in the program. The field might be for you to type in the reason why the client does not want to participate.

Additional information in this area might be:

- The frequency of care calls
- The information that should be covered on each call
- The materials that should be mailed to the client and when to mail them

Mailings/Materials

The software should have an area that keeps a running list of materials that have been sent to the client. Some software may have an option to either mail a hard copy of the material to the client or send it electronically through e-mail. Either way, the name of the item, the day it was ordered to be mailed (by you), and the day it was fulfilled (sent) should be documented.

Mailings are usually patient education handouts that can be for a variety of reasons. Some health plans/wellness programs have specific materials about immunizations, routine screening tests, and frequency of follow-up examinations that they want every person in the program to receive. Other programs will provide a list of materials available for a specific health problem. When on the phone with the client, you can pick and choose what material to have mailed to the client.

Remember to follow up during subsequent calls about any mailings. Ask the client if the material was received and if they have had a chance to read through it. Then ask if they have any questions.

Some health plans have alternative methods of providing teaching materials for individuals who are vision or hearing impaired. And, health plans today have teaching materials printed in the most common non-English languages. Be sure to select the best appropriate avenue when identifying teaching materials for your clients.

Health Plan/Disease Management Claims Data

To be complete, some software programs used by health plans and disease management programs have sections where claims data are listed. This section of the record would be for your information only and unable to be edited or changed. However, this information is extremely valuable. It can be used to validate the day surgery was performed and what type. It can be used to check when a prescribed medication was last filled and paid for by the health plan. Verifying diagnostic and laboratory testing can also be completed using this information.

Keep in mind, though, that claims data might not be documented in real time. This means there might be a few weeks or month lag time between the time of the event and the time the entry appears on the record. And if a claim is being disputed by the health plan, the information may never appear on the record. So in other words, this information is great to have if it is current, but it is not the most reliable method to validate or verify information.

LEARNING THE COMPUTERIZED DOCUMENTATION SYSTEM

Every nurse hired to provide telephonic care will be scheduled for orientation with the organization. The length of orientation can span a few days to several weeks; however, the average amount of time is 2 to 3 weeks. During orientation, you will be learning the organization's computerized documentation system.

For nurses new to telephonic care, this is the most stressful part of the job. The vast majority of nurses do not provide care and document care at the same time, which is what you are expected to do as a telephonic nurse. Your clinical trainer/staff development educator will most likely spend a great deal of time orienting you to the computer system and software used. You will probably have scenarios to practice inputting data and ideally have opportunities to role-play conversations while documenting.

Depending on the age of the nurse, the comfort level working with computers will differ. Nurses who are near the end of their careers may not have been exposed to computers at an early age. These nurses are considered digital immigrants and learning the use of a computer may be intimidating. Other nurses may have been raised on computers—or digital natives—and learning the software will be a breeze. But remember, talking and documenting at the same time is a skill that can be learned.

First, always remember that the client is the "patient" and not the computer. Keeping quiet on the telephone while you document is not acceptable. The client may ask "are you still there." Avoid saying things like "I'm sorry but my computer is running really slowly today." The client may wonder if the calls are worth the time waiting for the nurse to type everything that is said into the computer and stop accepting your calls.

Tips to Enhance Clinical Documentation

Everyone has hints, tips, and techniques to facilitate talking and typing at the same time. The following are just a few of the hints many nurses in the telephonic care field have used to improve their documentation speed and performance:

- *Practice exercises to improve hand–eye coordination.* This could be playing a game on the computer or using a handheld device like a smartphone.
- *Develop a pattern when documenting.* Some nurses float between medications, current health problems, and physical assessment data. If a client says he or she takes a medication for a health problem, the medication is documented, the health problem is documented, and the physical assessment information about the health problem is documented before moving to the next medication.
- *Print out dialogue that is most commonly used.* Until a comfort level is reached with talking on the telephone, some nurses find reading or referring to a guide sheet is helpful. This also ensures that nothing is accidentally skipped or missed when discussing the purpose of a program to a new enrollee.
- *Write the information down.* When all else fails and it is impossible at this time to keep up with the conversation flow and document at the same time, beginning telephonic nurses in the field have resorted to writing down the information during the call and then entering the information when the call ends. Keep in mind that this approach should be the exception. Nurses with a few months or years of telephonic care experience should not be writing down the content of every call and then documenting in the record. This takes considerable effort and time and increases the risk of violating privacy laws. Any client information that is written down should be destroyed appropriately. Throwing these bits of paper in the trash can under the desk is not acceptable.
- *Practice talking on the telephone and typing at the same time.* Some nurses have found it helpful to practice talking on the phone with family and friends at home while typing on a computer. Of course,

it is a bit easier to type dialogue than it might be to point, click, and find fields to document information in a software application; however, many nurses have used this technique to increase speed and reduce the length of time between asking a question and responding to the client during a call.

● *Give yourself time to learn.* Not every new telephonic nurse can hit the ground running at the expected level of performance. Give yourself time to learn. Ask questions. Expect to make mistakes.

AVOIDING THE MOST MAJOR MISTAKE OF ALL

This topic appears last in this chapter and has a separate heading for a very important reason. Every telephonic nurse has made this mistake at one point in their careers, and once you make it, you will never do it again. This mistake is forgetting to save information entered into the medical record.

Software applications created for telephonic care are not like the typical software that comes with home computers or portable devices. There is no "switch to flip" to set saving to occur at a predetermined length of time. The data most often must be physically saved to be recorded. The location of the SAVE button can be at the top or bottom of the screen. If you are scrolling through a screen, and the SAVE button is at the top, visually you will not see it unless you scroll back up to the top of the screen. The same can occur if the button is at the bottom of the screen and you did not have to scroll to the bottom to enter data. You can miss the SAVE button and your data will be lost.

Some nurses have placed a bright yellow note on the corner of their computer screens with the word SAVE in black letters to remind them to hit the SAVE button before changing screens or closing a client's medical record. Use whatever reminder that works the best for you.

At times, the data will not be automatically saved. You will have to exit the chart and open the chart again to see if the information you entered is "there." Until you feel secure that your information is being saved, taking an extra second or two to check is worth it. Imagine spending time on a welcome call and obtaining all required information only to learn a week later during the next call that the content from the welcome call was not saved. Some software programs may have a message that appears such as "do you want to save your data before exiting," but not all software has this feature. It is probably best to get used to frequently saving your inputted information early in your telephonic nursing career.

KEY POINTS

- There are many types of clinical computerized software packages for telephonic care.
- Your organization will have a specific software that is used that you will have to learn.
- You will not be expected to learn the software on your own but rather will have an orientation and time to practice.
- Develop a rhythm that works for you when documenting client information.
- Remember that the computer is not the patient.
- If entering data and talking at the same is challenging, spend some time at home practicing doing both.
- Develop tip sheets to keep yourself on track with content and expectations during care calls.
- Save your inputted information frequently.

CHAPTER 24

Tools for Telephonic Care

LEARNING OUTCOMES

Upon completion of this chapter, the nurse will:

1. Identify resource materials that would be beneficial when functioning in different nursing roles when providing telephonic care
2. Maintain a list of reputable and approved websites to access while providing telephonic care
3. Develop a practice pattern that maximizes success when providing telephonic care

RESOURCES

Regardless of the organization, health plan, or program through which you will be providing telephonic care, it is always wise to have resources available to help facilitate your care. It's not necessary to go out to buy tons of books and magazine subscriptions. A few choice items would be sufficient.

Resources that other telephonic nurses have found beneficial include:

- A current medical–surgical textbook
- A current manual of nursing practice
- A current nurses drug guide (not a *Physician's Desk Reference* [PDR])
- A current manual of diagnostic and laboratory tests
- A current *International Classification of Diseases, Revision 10* (ICD-10) and Current Procedural Terminology (CPT) coding guide
- Manual of medical nutrition

Most publishers consider "current" to be something that has been written with 5 years. Some nursing publishers realize, though, that things change more quickly than every 5 years and publish new editions every 2 to 3 years. For medical–surgical, nursing practice, diagnostic/laboratory tests, coding guides, and medical nutrition texts, updating every 5 years would be sufficient. Drug guides, however, should be updated yearly. New medications are being developed rapidly, and a drug guide that is 5 years old is considered outdated.

The organization should provide the following materials for all staff:

- Policy and procedure manual
- Guidelines for placing welcome calls
- Guidelines for placing care calls
- Guidelines to enroll members into a program
- Guidelines to disenroll members from a program
- Specific guidelines to address disease management program expectations
- Specific guidelines to address wellness program expectations
- Specific guidelines to support various nursing roles

VARIOUS NURSING ROLES IN TELEPHONIC CARE

Nurses are accustomed to having expertise in different areas of health care, and telephonic care is not an exception. Depending on the health plan or disease management or wellness program, nurses may be designated or assigned different care responsibilities. Types of different roles for telephonic nurses include:

- Posthospital care
- Case management
- Welcome calls
- Care calls
- Reminder calls

Posthospital Care

Nurses who are assigned to provide posthospital care calls will be spending a large amount of time on each call. The purpose of these calls is to:

- Find out the reason for the hospitalization
- What occurred while hospitalized such as surgery or change in treatments

- Any changes to medications
- Next health care provider appointment
- Future plan such as additional surgery
- Update current health status
- Update diagnostic and laboratory tests

Once all of the posthospitalization calls are completed, the nurse may be assigned to contact clients in another care category.

Case Management

Oftentimes telephonic organizations, health plans, and disease/wellness programs will have nurses who are certified case managers provide telephonic care calls. These nurses will conduct case management activities to include making referrals and contacting the health plan and health care provider.

Welcome Calls

A welcome call introduces a client to the telephonic program. Of all of the different types of care calls, this one is probably the most important. This is the client's first exposure to the process of telephonic care, and the way the program is introduced and the manner in which it is introduced depends on the nurse's skill and comfort level.

Some organizations/health plans/disease management plans provide a cheat sheet or guide sheet to be used during the welcome call. This is to ensure that the client verbally receives all essential information before going forward in the program. As was mentioned in a previous chapter, the health plan or disease or wellness management program will most likely mail the client information about being enrolled in the program. The welcome call should occur after the materials have arrived and the client has had an opportunity to review them.

Unfortunately, this is not always the case and the nurse might find that a client has no idea what the program is or why they have been enrolled. In these situations, the nurse has to supplement information while encouraging the client to participate.

Care Calls

Care calls are those that occur after the welcome call. The frequency of calls will depend on the client's health status and willingness to accept the calls. Some care calls are appropriate to make every week. Clients who are in the middle of an exacerbation of a chronic health problem or are experiencing a new health problem would qualify for weekly calls. The intention for these calls is to help identify any new issues, bring them to the attention of the health care provider, and strive to prevent the client from needing hospitalization.

Once the acute problem has subsided, the frequency of care calls can be reduced to biweekly. For some organizations, every 2 weeks is a standard for what is considered "routine" care calls.

Clients in wellness programs who are not experiencing any new or different health problems may receive calls every month. The option always exists to contact these clients more frequently, but once-a-month calls are usually sufficient to prevent the client from developing a new health problem or needing hospitalization.

Reminder Calls

These are calls that are made on a monthly or quarterly basis and serve to remind the client that "something" needs to be done. Reasons for reminder calls include:

- Quarterly hemoglobin A1c levels to be checked
- Seasonal influenza vaccination recommended
- Annual eye examination recommended
- Biannual podiatrist examination recommended
- Annual urine albumin level recommended

These calls are in addition to, and not instead of, the other types of calls.

OTHER RESOURCES

At times, you might need to research a new treatment or medication that is not identified in your resources books. This is when you might have to access the Internet. The use of the Internet in organizations is typically limited to work-related searches. Some organizations may screen searches and only present those that have been approved. Other organizations may block the use of the Internet altogether.

There is value in having access to the Internet during telephonic care calls. If a client asks a question or mentions a new medication and has questions about the side effects, you can do a quick medication search and provide the information immediately to the client. Sometimes, a client may be experiencing an adverse reaction to a new medication and think a new problem is developing. A quick Internet search could allay the client's anxieties and provide the support that you need for the client to contact the health care provider immediately.

Remember that the Internet is a large toolbox that contains all types of information. Not all information is valid and in some situations, could be harmful if followed. You will need to learn which Internet sources are reliable and which ones to avoid.

In general, any Internet address that ends in .gov is considered reliable. The sites might be from:

- The National Institutes of Health (https://www.nih.gov)
- Medline (U.S. National Library of Medicine; https://www.nlm.nih.gov/bsd/pmresources.html)
- Medline Plus (https://www.nlm.nih.gov/medlineplus)
- Centers for Medicare and Medicaid Services (https://www.cms.gov)
- Centers for Disease Control and Prevention (http://www.cdc.gov)
- State health departments

Other reliable sites include:

- The World Health Organization (http://www.who.int/en)
- American Heart Association (http://www.heart.org)
- American Lung Association (http://www.lung.org)
- American Diabetes Association (http://www.diabetes.org)

Usually, any site that is sponsored by a national organization is considered reliable.

Maybe you need to search for information that is not mainstream, and you receive a list of websites that you are not sure if they are reliable. A few things that you can do to determine the reliability of a website include:

- Look for the name and credentials of the person who wrote the material or article
- Look to see if the article was printed in a reputable journal in addition to being posted online

- Look to see if the material has a "last reviewed" date; this usually appears at the bottom of the page

Avoid websites that end in .blog or are Wordpress sponsored. These are individual pages published by all kinds of people who may or may not have the credentials to write about the topic. Another website that you might receive when doing a search is About.com. This website is written by individuals who are freelance writers and who may not have any health care experience. Wikipedia is another source with questionable reliability of the content. Even though Wikipedia often lists resources at the bottom of the article, the resources may be questionable.

Some organizations may request that information published on drug company websites not be shared with clients. There is a tendency for drug company websites to only provide positive information about the medication, and potential side or adverse effects cannot be found. There are other reputable sites to learn information about recent or new medications that can be used instead.

You do not need to purchase any subscriptions to access reliable content on the Internet. If you do a search and an article appears that provides only the abstract, the site is expecting you to pay for the rest of the article. Unless your organization has a subscription to the site, click off of the article and return to your search list and find another resource to use.

At times, a client may have conducted his or her own Internet search and has questions about something that was read online. To help the client discern if the content is reliable:

- Ask the client for the website address
- Access the information
- Take a few minutes and review the information
- Make a decision if the content is valid

Some clients are unable to determine if information on the Internet is reliable and may believe whatever is written, regardless of the author or the source.

PRACTICE PATTERNS

If you asked 10 nurses who provide telephonic care how they approach their calls, you would receive 10 different responses. And, they would all be correct. There is no "one right way" to make the calls. You will have to use the trial and error approach to figure out what works the best for you.

Some telephonic nurses have had to develop "the gift of gab" to be successful. This means mastering the art of "small talk" such as:

- Asking how the weather is, where the client is located
- Finding out if the client has any pets and their names
- If the client has children/grandchildren and when they will be visiting
- The client's interests and hobbies
- What the client does or did while employed
- If the client has lived in the same community for many years
- If there are any special occasions coming up in the client's life such as a birthday, family wedding, graduation, or baby showers
- What sports the client has an interest in and the names of teams the client follows

Of course, the purpose of care calls is not to "touch base" and "catch up" with current events in the client's life; however, being able to "chat" about nonhealth-related things personalizes the telephone call. These bits and pieces of conversation strengthen the nurse–client relationship. It demonstrates that you care enough to ask about a family member, a pet, or an upcoming event. You are not just some nurse that calls every now and then to ask what laboratory work was done, what medications were changed, and if the client lost any weight. You will become "my nurse" who "calls me to make sure that I'm doing ok" and "answers questions that I have." You will become the nurse who is called immediately after a health care provider's appointment to report any changes in medications and the results of laboratory work. Instead of the client waiting for you to call, the client can't wait to call you with the information and share their news.

CHEAT SHEETS

Some organizations and nurses have created "cheat sheets" to be used during calls. These sheets might be:

- Printouts of the computer screens and fields
- Suggested dialogue to use during specific calls
- Specific information that should be shared on specific calls

- Names and telephone numbers of support groups or other resources within a client's community
- Names and telephone numbers of the health plan or disease management or wellness program
- Names and telephone numbers of national agencies
- New updates to any information that should be shared during care calls
- Names, telephone numbers, and extensions of any health care professionals that have been identified by the health plan to use for specific situations

These cheat sheets are invaluable and should be kept ready at hand to refer to at any time.

At times, nurses who have been providing telephonic care for extended periods of time may have created shortcuts or work-arounds that can help with documenting in the computer software. These documents are worth their weight in gold. Collect them whenever they are offered and study them to see if they can help you with your documentation and care calls.

KEY POINTS

- Having resources available when conducting care calls saves time, facilitates the calls, and provides clients with "real-time" requested information.
- Use the resources provided by the organization. Keep them in a book or binder on your desk for easy access.
- Realize that the Internet is a tool and that not all of the information is valid.
- Learn to identify Internet resources that are the most valid from those that are opinion or blog pieces.
- Think of ways to keep your client engaged during care calls. This might mean talking about something totally unrelated to health or listening to them complain about a noisy neighbor.
- Never underestimate the value of cheat sheets. The ideal telephonic care environment embraces lifelong learning. There is something new to learn every day when practicing telephonic nursing. Look forward to learning new things and then sharing the information with others.

CHAPTER 25

Work Environments

LEARNING OUTCOMES

Upon completion of this chapter, the nurse will:

1. Explain the advantages and disadvantages of different work environments for providing telephonic care
2. Analyze the work environment that would best suit the nurse's personality and work processes
3. Strive to achieve the best possible work environment to support client care

ENVIRONMENTS

In general, there are only two types of work environments for telephonic care: a call center and home. All telephonic care organizations started by using the call center format.

Call Center

A call center is a big office, with cubicles or desks, lined up in rows. Depending on the size of the office, 50 to 100 desk spaces could be in the center. Each nurse has a desk space, or cubicle, that typically includes:

- A desktop
- A telephone
- A computer and peripherals (keyboard, mouse)
- A few desk drawers
- A bookshelf
- A trash can
- A desk chair

It is up to you to try to make this work environment as comfortable and useful as possible. Some nurses bring pictures of their family and pets to place on their desk. Others might have small plants to add a bit of "green" to the environment. Unless there was a policy stating otherwise, nurses have been known to bring their goldfish with them to work and watch them swim happily while the nurse makes telephonic calls.

You will need desk supplies. This is different from needing a stethoscope, rolls of paper tape, and syringes to provide care. Supplies to set up your desk would include:

- Tablets/paper
- Pens/pencils
- Paper clips
- Push pins
- Binders
- Hole punch
- Highlighter markers
- File folders
- Envelopes
- Tape
- Calendar

Oftentimes, the organization will have a room set aside for supplies to set up a desk space. Preparing the desk is usually one of the last things done at the end of the orientation period and before actual care calls are being made.

In time you might find that you need additional items to make your work area more comfortable to enhance your productivity. You might need:

- A chair pillow
- A small desk lamp
- A clock

The telephone system might take some getting used to when beginning to provide telephonic care. Holding a telephone handset up to your ear for hours at a time can be tiring. Because of this, most organizations provide headsets. This is a device that has a receiver over one ear and a tube that is used to talk through. Some nurses find headsets uncomfortable at first but that quickly goes away. The alternative is holding a handset, which can be challenging if trying to type, talk, and balance a handset between the ear and shoulder at the same time.

There are advantages to working in a call center for telephonic care. Some of these advantages include:

- Having other people with which to discuss client care situations
- Feeling like a member of a team
- Having access to a photocopy machine
- Having many different resources available
- Having someone available to help if the computer or telephone breaks

Other advantages to providing telephonic care that a nurse who has worked providing direct client care may not realize include:

- Not wearing uniforms anymore
- Not having to prepare for report
- Not having to give the next shift report
- Not having to count narcotics
- Not having to document on several assigned clients at the same time
- Not having to provide medications, treatments, or therapies at specific times
- Not having to call physicians to report laboratory values or take verbal orders
- Not having to rotate shifts or work a "double" because of staffing issues

The client situations in telephonic care are different as well. Remember, the client is at home and you will not need to:

- Measure or evaluate vital signs
- Monitor intake and output
- Prepare and administer medications
- Prepare, administer, and monitor intravenous fluids or blood transfusions
- Flush multiple tubes and drains
- Follow up with tasks delegated to other staff members
- Work mandatory overtime to cover other staffing issues

This change in the type of care provided may be unsettling for some nurses new to telephonic care. Give yourself time to learn the position, and in time you will see the value and importance of providing care using this approach.

Home

Over the years, some telephonic organizations have downsized their office spaces and decentralized the nursing staff to work at home. For some nurses, this was the reason to seek a telephonic nursing care position. Most nurses, however, have to first work in the call center to learn the position before being considered qualified to provide care through a home office.

Setting up a home office can be overwhelming at first. Things to consider include:

- Where the office will be located in the home
- Responsibility for the telephone
- Responsibility for the computer
- Ensuring the environment is secure to adhere to privacy laws
- Process to destroy client personal health information
- Process to call for help if equipment breaks
- Process to call for help if an unusual client situation occurs

A person may desire to work at home but find that he or she does not really like it. The home becomes a place of work, and there is a tendency to be "always working." On the other hand, a person might think that because the office is "right next door," there is no rush to get to work.

Working at home takes dedication and discipline. It also takes a person who is intrinsically motivated to complete projects and tasks. The organization will most likely send an employee out to your home to help set up the equipment and make sure that the office space meets privacy and legal expectations. You will also most likely make telephone calls after logging in to a telephone network system. Be advised that your time on the telephone will be documented. A home office is to perform work and will be monitored.

Having the option to work at home has its advantages:

- No need to "dress up" to go to work
- Not having to drive through traffic or inclement weather to get to work
- No issues with parking or public transportation to get to work
- Reduced expenses for transportation and meals away from the home
- Having a comfortable working environment

Even though you might be identified as a nurse who works from the home, you may still need to "go into the office" periodically for meetings, events, or updates. Consider going into the main office as a bonus day. You will have an opportunity to catch up with other friends and colleagues, most likely learn information about the organization and health plan, and have a chance to legitimately get away from your desk. Some organizations plan a day a month for the home workers to come into the office. During this day, the colleagues attend a company-wide meeting, have small meetings with their team and manager, participate in continuing education, and share a meal with friends. It becomes an event to look forward to instead of something that has to be done.

IDEAL WORK ENVIRONMENT

No one can determine the best work environment for someone else. It depends on the nurse's personality, temperament, and comfort level. Things to consider when determining the best work environment include:

Call Center	Home Office
• Likes to be around other people • Needs others to support motivation • Likes to discuss client care issues with others • Likes to work in an environment that can be noisy at times • Looks forward to talking with friends about nonwork-related things • Enjoys commuting to work every day • Lives in an environment that supports a daily work commute • Does not have adequate room or location in the home to set up a home office • Cannot ensure that other family members will not interrupt during hours of work • Has limited professional resources to use for care calls • Likes to share meals with others at work	• Likes to work alone or in isolation • Intrinsically motivated to accomplish tasks • Likes to work in a relatively quiet environment • Prefers to meet with friends outside of the work environment • Has challenges with a daily commute • Lives in an environment that does not support an easy daily commute such as frequent inclement weather or access to public transportation is limited • Has adequate room or space in the home to set up a home office • Can ensure that family members will not interrupt during hours of work • Has adequate professional resources to use for care calls • Has no issue with eating a meal alone

WORK ISSUES

The ideal work environment does not exist. It is up to every nurse to create an environment where calls can be made, care provided, and documentation completed so that at the end of the day, you feel satisfaction in accomplishing the organization's goals and helped improve the health of your clients.

Working in a call center, realize that others will most likely hear your conversations. For some nurses, this could be uncomfortable, but keep in mind that you can hear the other nurses too and you might just pick up a few words or phrases that you could use when talking with your clients.

Your organization will most likely have a leadership or management team in place. Similar to being assigned to work on a team or on a particular unit in a direct care facility, telephonic nurses will also be divided or placed into teams. Some organizations refer to these as work groups.

Your "team leader" or "manager" will be monitoring your performance. This could be in the form of sitting with you while making care calls or listening in on calls from a remote location. Afterward, you will be provided with feedback. Depending on the organization, expect to have these monitoring calls completed at least every quarter in a calendar year. This information is used to complete your annual performance appraisal and is a method to identify any learning needs that you may have to improve your performance.

As the organization grows and additional nurses are hired, you might be asked to serve as a mentor for a new employee. Because the new employee most likely has been in orientation, your role as a mentor is to demonstrate "putting it all together" when making care calls. There are telephone devices that can be used (double headsets) so that both you and the new employee can be on the telephone call with the client at the same time—however, only one person can talk at a time. The use of double headsets gives the employee an opportunity to observe firsthand the flow of a call, the use of the computer software, and the types of interventions provided.

When preparing to make calls, you will have to log into the computer system and the dialer. The dialer is a separate computer system that prepares and creates lists of client telephone numbers to be called for a particular reason or time of day. Your team leader/manager will tell you which "bucket" of calls to log into at the beginning of your work day. When you are ready to start providing care and making calls, you tell the dialer electronically that you are "ready" and it will queue up the next call and begin dialing the number. At the same time, the client's medical record will present on your computer screen. There really is not much time for you to go through a client's record before starting the call, so it is essential for you to become as comfortable as possible with the clinical documentation system early in your work career with the organization.

Once the call is completed and the client hangs up, you will also need to hang up through the dialer. At this time, you can spend a few extra minutes adding documentation and ensuring that everything that was completed and discussed is documented. Prior to telling the dialer that you are ready for the next client call, save your entered information. You repeat this process until all of the calls in the assigned "bucket" have been completed.

The dialer becomes your daily monitor. You log into the dialer, you tell the dialer when you are ready to take calls, you tell the dialer when you are going on a "break" so that calls do not come to your telephone when you are not there, and you log out of the dialer at the end of the work day.

Some nurses may feel that the dialer restricts their care because it measures the length of time on the calls. Other nurses learn to ignore the dialer and focus solely on the care the client needs at that present time. Your team leader/manager will explain the purpose of the dialer for the organization and if the amount of time spent on a call is of importance. For posthospitalization, welcome, and routine care calls, the amount of time spent on a call may be great. For reminder calls, the calls will be short. It really just depends on the purpose of the call and the response that you receive once the client is contacted.

If you are working for an organization that has several contracts for health plans or disease management programs, there might be times when the volume of required calls for a particular day is extreme. These are usually program "kick-off" days, which means the organization is officially beginning to provide telephonic care to a set of enrolled clients. The leadership team members might be walking around the call center during these days, observing how the work flow is going with the nurses and periodically reporting the teams' successes in contacting the newly enrolled clients. Some organizations mark this day as a celebration for the organization and may provide some sort of congratulatory treat for all staff such as providing lunch or having an afternoon snack in the breakroom for all to enjoy.

Even with the "perceived" restrictions imposed by the dialer and the periodic expectations to reach out and contact as many clients as possible on specific days, working as a telephonic nurse can be a joyful experience. The camaraderie that develops between team members is unlike any other direct care work environment. There is a feeling of family when at work, and everyone pitches in to help achieve the organization's daily goals.

KEY POINTS

- There are two types of work environments for telephonic care.
- The call center is the most prevalent type.
- The option to work at home may be offered after demonstrating competence providing telephonic care in a call center environment.
- There are advantages and disadvantages to each type of work environment.
- The organization provides support with both types of work environments.
- Nurses personalize their call center spaces.
- The dialer is a tool that prepares, presents, and monitors the volume of care calls made.

CHAPTER 26

Issues and Solutions

Upon completion of this chapter the nurse will:

1. Summarize different issues that can arise when making telephonic care calls
2. Brainstorm approaches to overcome issues that can arise when making telephonic care calls
3. Realize that telephonic care has a unique set of challenges

ISSUES AND SOLUTIONS

Similar to providing direct care, telephonic care has a few issues and challenges. These issues can be categorized as being related to people, paper, or processes.

People

Clients

The issues with people occur at different levels. The most obvious is with the client. Clients are not always willing or interested in participating in a telephonic care program. They may have a variety of excuses ranging from "I have a doctor" to "what kind of care are you going to give me over the telephone?" Additional issues are provided next with suggestions to respond to the client.

Issue	Response
How much is this going to cost me?	This is included as a benefit with your health plan.
I didn't ask for this benefit so I'm paying for something that I don't want or need.	Questions about your benefits should be directed to your health plan. Do you have the telephone number to contact them directly?
So you didn't cut it as a real nurse, huh?	Telephonic care is a valid care delivery approach. I have provided direct care to clients but choose to practice this method now.
Why are you calling me so much? What do you want?	I am calling to introduce you to a program that you are enrolled in through your health plan.
If you want to know anything about my health, call my doctor.	This program contacts the client directly. Our contact with physicians is through the client.
You always bother me when I'm eating.	What would be a better time of day to reach you?
Here—talk to my wife.	First I need permission from you to talk with any other family member about your health.
Who are you? Where's the other nurse I talked with 2 weeks ago?	The other nurse is unavailable at this time. I work with the other nurse, and we support each other's clients.
Is that all you do, ask questions?	It might seem like I'm asking a lot of questions, but the answers help me decide the best care for you.
I'm not feeling good today. Will you call and tell my doctor that I need an appointment?	Our contact with the doctors is through you. We can end the call now so you can contact your doctor to make an appointment.
I don't want these calls or need these calls. If I need any help, I'll go to the emergency room.	That's the purpose of these calls—to make sure you don't need to use the emergency room for an immediate problem.

(continued)

(continued)

Issue	Response
I'm home now. Come on over and we can talk.	Thank you for the offer, but we are not located in the same state. Our care is provided over the telephone.
So you're like a home care nurse, but you don't see the patient?	A home care nurse will check your immediate needs and provide direct care. We help you prevent additional problems so you won't need to be hospitalized.
I'm tired. Call me tomorrow morning. CLICK	(Change the day and best time to call to reflect the next day.)
How did you get my phone number?	The information regarding your telephone number is provided through your health plan.
All you want me to do is to make appointments to see my doctor every 3 months. Do you know that I have to pay $20 every time I go see him? How's that a benefit?	It's important to have regular checkups with your health care provider about health problems. That's the reason we encourage keeping to a routine visit schedule.
You people are all alike. All you do is hound me to (quit smoking/stop drinking/lose weight).	Changing your behavior with (smoking cessation/reduced alcohol intake/weight management) is to help you improve your health so you won't get sick and need to be in the hospital.

As you spend more time with clients, you might learn of a few additional situations to add to this list.

Health Plan/Disease Management/Wellness Program

At times, you may have to talk with members of the client's health plan or program to have information changed or validated. For example, a client adamantly denies having a health problem, yet the client still presents in the call queue with the problem. You change the information in the computer documentation system and save the information, but the next day the client is still identified as needing to be contacted for the health problem. It seems the only way to successfully disenroll the client is to call the health plan to have the client physically removed from the health plan's end.

When you finally get through to someone at the health plan, the person tells you that there are several claims for the health problem. You have already talked about the testing with the client and the reason being to rule out the health problem. The client is not pre-scribed any medication for the health problem and is not going to be receiving any treatments. The health plan individual may not be happy with you; however, do not give up—expect to have the client disenrolled.

Keep in mind that people who are working for the health plan most often field calls from disgruntled enrollees. When trying to understand a charge or a claim, the enrollee can become angry. Health plan employees may sound harsh when contacted, which could be because they are expecting another argument. There is no need to argue. Disenrolling the client from the plan is saving the health plan money and not the organization you work for.

Coworkers

Unfortunately, the profession of nursing has a history of bullying and incivility. This might even be a reason for someone to leave bedside care and seek employment as a telephonic nurse. Even so, there might be situations in which incivility rears its ugly head in the telephonic care environment.

This information is not being provided as a warning but rather to provide an explanation. At times, the organization may be chal-lenged to complete a large amount of work in a limited period of time. The number of staff available to provide care might not be suf-ficient to achieve the care call goals. The leadership staff have been notified that the health plan/disease management/wellness pro-gram expects a report showing the number of enrollees contacted and the anticipated day/time for the next call. Dialer reports are being run hourly to measure the success of the staff in meeting the expectation, and the leadership staff are wringing their hands instead of cracking a whip.

Now, bring this situation to the telephonic nurse level. The nurse is in a Welcome call dialer queue for individuals with diabetes. The health plan expects all demographics to be updated, medications entered, and the physical assessment started. In addition, at least two patient teaching tools should be ordered before ending the call. In order to meet the organization's goal for the client contacts for the day, each one of your calls should last no longer than 6 minutes so that each nurse contacts 10 clients every hour.

An immediate knee-jerk reaction is "this is impossible," and you might be right. Sometimes it takes 6 minutes to convince a client to participate in the program, even before any validation of demographics occurs. So, right now, the health plan is putting pressure on the organization, the leadership staff is stressed and studying dialer reports, and you, the nurse providing the calls, are told to stop talking so much and just get the information the health plan needs now. Someone is going to react negatively to all of the stress.

What you can do should this occur is this: stay calm, analyze how much time you are spending on "small talk," and possibly begin the call with the client with a statement such as "I won't keep you longer than 5 minutes today. Our next call can be longer, but I don't want to take up too much of your time." This sets the expectation with the client that the call will be short. You can move through the demographics. Then ask about medications such as "Because you are in our diabetes program, do you take insulin or another medication for that every day?" After you get the important medication for the primary health problem you can ask "are there any other medications that you take such as something for your heart or blood pressure?" Asking these direct questions keeps the client on track. You can end the medication portion of the call by asking a general question such as "is there anything else that you take daily such as acetaminophen or vitamin supplements?" Within a few minutes, the medication list is complete.

This leaves starting the assessment and ordering patient teaching tools. A good opening for this might be "do you have any other health problems or symptoms that you experience every day?" This gives the client the opportunity to focus on what is the most important to them. Depending on the answer, you can document this information in the appropriate area on the physical assessment. In preparation to end the call, you can then ask "how about if I send you some information to help you manage your diabetes? This would be a general fact sheet with some pointers that you might find helpful. And while I'm at it I'll add another sheet that focuses on the type of medication you take. Because you will get these materials in about a week, how about if I schedule your next call for 2 weeks from now? That way you will get the material and have a chance to look it over before I call back."

Keep in mind that this dialogue is only a suggestion; however, it has been used successfully by other telephonic nurses.

Even when everyone is doing their best during a stressful time, tempers can flair. One nurse overhears someone else say something that is incorrect or was supposed to be changed a week ago. Bickering occurs and everyone stops talking to hear what's going on. Unless you are directly involved, stay away from the problem. Listen to what the issue is to make sure that you are not making the same error but otherwise do not get involved. The team leader will intervene and settle the situation. The nurses involved may be testy with each other for a while, but in time that will fade.

The amount of bullying and incivility that occurs in a telephonic care environment is minute compared to the extent of the issue with bedside care providers. Knowing that it can occur and the reasons why helps prevent it from happening in the first place.

Paper

Even though the work of telephonic care occurs with a telephone and computer, you will accumulate a large amount of paper resources. You will have your orientation manual, copies of health plan guide sheets, samples of patient teaching tools (or possibly copies of every tool), cheat sheets, lists of resources, and contact telephone numbers. There is no possible way for you to miss something, right? Not necessarily.

Work in a telephonic environment is fluid. Things change. The health plan adds something and takes something else away. The organization adds something to a policy but deletes steps from a procedure. A new feature is added to the computer documentation system, and cheat sheets are missing a few steps. In other words, all of the paper needs to be updated.

The team leader makes copies of the changed pages with the intention to distribute them to all team staff members. A situation occurs, and the new pages are placed on a desk. Hours later, the team leader returns to the desk to find the pages missing or moved. Who received the updates? Who still needs the updates? Is there time to make more copies to distribute before the updates take effect? What about the people who work part time and won't get the updates until the weekend? Who is going to help them understand the updates? What should be done first?

Static (paper) resources do not fit well with a fluid environment because of the frequency of changes. The organization might implement another approach: place all updates on a shared computer file, and then send a group e-mail to all staff informing of the changed document. The staff can then either keep the file on the computer hard drive or print it out to replace the other static page that is outdated.

For major policy or procedure changes, each manual should be updated with the correct information; however, every staff member does not need a personal copy. A list of the changes to keep the staff informed is sufficient.

Processes

This brings us to the final issue that can create challenges in the telephonic care environment—processes. Process changes are the major reason why the paper issues occur. Processes are explanations of how to "do something" or the "work" of providing telephonic care. Processes are reviewed and practiced in orientation. Processes are mastered when working with the computer documentation system. Processes are essential because they standardize actions to improve efficiency and effectiveness.

When a process fails, things can quickly get out of hand. Someone needs to take the time to go through the process to see which step or steps are out of sync or causing issues. Then, new steps need to be identified to replace those that no longer work. Once the new steps are added, the process needs to be tested to make sure that no other issues occur. Finally, the new process is complete and ready to be distributed to all for immediate implementation.

Depending on the process, identifying, revising, and retraining can take hours, days, or even weeks. While the process is being improved or changed, tempers can flair and anxiety builds. Staff become concerned, and team leaders are not happy.

One way to reduce the effects of process issues is to expect them to change. Many nurses have said "I no sooner learn how to do something when it changes and I have to learn how to do it all over again." This is the nature of telephonic care. Fluid environments are constantly changing. And you might not feel like you have mastered anything for quite some time. Providing care in this type of environment is not like mastering the preparation and provision of injections or calibrating intravenous fluids in a flash. Those skills do not change. However, the intricacies of telephonic care can and will change. But, what does not change is the goal of contacting clients to discuss health needs and approaches to maximize wellness and meet personal goals.

HANDLING THE STRESS

Remember the days when clients were falling out of bed, intravenous lines were being pulled out, and doctors were yelling at you because orders weren't completed yet? Your worst day as a telephonic nurse does not even come close to the stresses of a bedside nurse. Remember this when you become anxious and wonder if you made the right decision to become a telephonic nurse.

You made the right decision. You are:

- Providing care to a tremendous number of people with a huge potential impact on their health status
- Helping control the cost of health care by early identification of health problems
- Empowering clients to discuss their health needs with the health care provider
- Helping reshape the health care industry

Congratulations! Now go make some care calls!

KEY POINTS

- The major issues or challenges with telephonic care are categorized as related to people, paper, or processes.
- Not every client welcomes telephonic care. You may need to convince some clients to participate.
- Work environment situations can make staff members testy. Do your best and focus on what you need to accomplish.
- The amount of paper you need to do your job may be overwhelming. And, the papers may and will change.
- Processes can and will change. Knowing this in advance will help reduce any work-related stress.
- If discouragement strikes, remember your days working as a bedside nurse.
- View your efforts as an integral part of the health care industry.

CHAPTER 27

The Nurse as Client

LEARNING OUTCOMES

Upon completion of this chapter, the nurse will:

1. Review behaviors to maximize personal strengths and capabilities
2. Strategize ways to ensure personal health
3. Consider adopting the behavior of "practicing what I preach"

PERSONAL CARE

The title of this chapter was selected to get your attention. This chapter is for you—the telephonic nurse. It is very easy to fall into patterns that are harmful to your health, particularly when moving from a position of direct care provider to one of telephonic nurse. Probably, one of the major issues is that of weight management.

Weight Management

Most everyone has heard of the "freshman 15": a first-year college student gains 15 pounds because of late-night eating and other indulgences. Well, there is a similar phenomenon in telephonic care. It is called the "telephonic 20." Yes, you read it correctly. There is the potential to gain 20 pounds just from changing jobs.

How can this happen? It is really quite simple. As a direct care provider, you were moving constantly. The only time you might have been seated was to document and even that was interrupted by answering call lights, taking phone calls, or rushing to provide a pain medication before going into report. You were expending a great deal of physical energy and might not always had a chance to have a meal.

Your caloric expenditure was equal to or possibly even less than what you were taking in.

Then you applied and were accepted for a position as a telephonic nurse. In your new job, you drive (or use some other method of transportation) and park in a lot next to the main office. You might have to walk a few hundred steps to the elevator. Then you walk to your desk (or cubicle), hang up your coat, put away your personal items, get a cup of coffee (or something similar), and sit down at your desk to begin your workday.

Calls are presenting to your desktop and you are on a roll. Before you know it 2 hours have passed, and you put yourself on "break" through the dialer. You walk to the break room (or staff kitchen) and chat with a few colleagues, read through a new posting on the bulletin board, and pour another cup of coffee before going back to your desk.

You resume working until your lunch break. You tell the dialer you are on lunch, and you talk with other team members and share a pizza that was delivered a few minutes ago. The time flies, and you get back to your desk and resume your workday.

During an afternoon break, you walk to the photocopy machine to make a copy of a cheat sheet for a new employee and then return to your desk for a few more hours of care calls before the end of the day.

You log out of the dialer, collect your personal items, saunter past a few colleagues' cubicles, and chat as you work your way to the elevator and walk the few hundred steps back to your car, where you proceed to sit, again, for the drive home.

The amount of exercise you receive as a telephonic nurse is equivalent to less than an hour as a direct care provider. And, if you do not adjust your physical activity when you are not at work or alter your eating plan, the telephonic 20 will occur in record time.

This situation leads to the next issue that telephonic nurses experience: the hazards of immobility.

Hazards of Immobility

Every nurse knows what can occur to a client who has been placed on bed rest while hospitalized:

- Muscle atrophy
- Skin breakdown

- Reduced respiratory excursion
- Pooling of blood in the lower extremities
- Sluggish abdominal organ function (i.e., constipation)
- Potential for renal calculi formation
- Hip contractures
- Muscle tension

As a telephonic nurse, you now are at risk for these same hazards. However, do not be hasty and hand in your letter of resignation. There are a few lifestyle changes that you can make to combat these hazards. And you might just recognize these approaches because they are very similar (if not identical) to the ones you use to encourage your clients to perform.

Exercise/Activity

Telephonic nurses have to plan or schedule activity. Because you will be sitting for most, if not all, of the workday, you will need to get exercise or activity some other way. Some suggestions include:

- Parking a bit farther away from the main office door so that you have to walk more to and from the car
- Taking a brief walk during a break or after lunch
- Changing the type of foods eaten during breaks and lunch
- Drinking more water instead of convenience drinks (like soda)
- Using hand weights while talking to clients (yes, telephonic nurses have lifted a few pounds of hand weights while waiting for a client call to connect)
- Planning to walk the dog the first thing in the morning and again at the end of the day

For those telephonic nurses who work at home, the challenge is even more acute. Additional physical activity losses for these nurses include:

- Walking to and from the car
- Walking to an elevator
- Walking around an office

And because there are no interruptions or other people around, the telephonic nurse working at home can easily sit for hours without moving anything beyond a few hand muscles for typing and the facial muscles to talk.

Nurses working at home really have to make major adjustments to prevent the telephonic 20 from multiplying and allay the hazards of immobility. Plan to:

- Get up and walk or stand at your desk every hour
- Perform something physical several times a day (make the bed, take out the trash, walk the dog, walk up and down the steps, pull weeds in the garden)
- Stand more at the end of your workday
- Increase activity on days off from work (not encouraging to become a weekend warrior but be aware of the need to increase activity)

Listen to what you say to your clients

Everyone has heard the phrase "do as I say, not as I do." This applies to the telephonic nurse. Every telephonic nurse has an anthology of tips and techniques to help clients improve their health status. These tips are usually prefaced by phrases such as:

- "Have you considered . . ."
- "What about trying . . ."
- "How about if you . . ."

It is now time for the phrases to be used on you. For preventing weight gain:

- Have you considered changing your food choices?
- What about using low-fat/low-calorie food items?
- How about if you substituted one treat for a piece of fruit each day?

For increasing activity:

- Have you considered using a treadmill, stationary bike, or joining a neighborhood fitness center?
- What about trying to take a walk during your midmorning, lunch, and afternoon breaks?
- How about if you did a few sit-ups or lunges while waiting for the pot to boil when making dinner?

Recognize health problems

Many people have said that health care providers make the worst patients because they know too much or they deny what they are experiencing. This is also true for the telephonic nurse.

You will be assessing clients, day in and day out, and can easily recognize a symptom as being a precursor to a disease process but will overlook or ignore the same symptom in yourself. This is called basic human nature; however, you have all of the tools right in front of you.

If you suspect something is amiss, do not ignore it. Take your own advice and seek medical attention. Call your doctor for routine checkups. See your dentist. Get your eyes examined. Make sure you have routine diagnostic tests done. Be as kind to yourself as you are to your clients. You are the most important person, to you. And, you deserve the care.

STRESS MANAGEMENT

There are various levels of stress. Mild stress causes a bit of anxiety. Moderate stress increases motivation and expends energy. Extreme stress, though, can be paralyzing. You need to avoid extreme stress.

What causes stress as a telephonic nurse?

- Unrealistic expectations
- Not giving yourself enough time to learn
- Not realizing that telephonic nursing is different than any other type of care you may have provided in your career
- Taking yourself too seriously

So what can you do to counter the effects of stress caused by telephonic nursing care?

Cultivate Friendships

Employment with one organization needs to end before starting a job with a new organization. When leaving a previous place of employment, you are leaving behind friends and colleagues that you might have worked with and established relationships with for years. When starting a new position, those friends and colleagues won't be there to see and talk with you every day. You are essentially starting over.

The other nurses in your orientation class will become your "instant" friends. You are all starting the job at the same time and have the same level of knowledge and expertise. The sense of camaraderie and feeling that we are "all in this together" creates an instant support group for the new employee.

Once orientation concludes, you receive your team assignment. Because other employees from your orientation class may or may not be on your new team, your support group has just vanished, and you find yourself feeling alone, again. But this will not last. Telephonic nurses have an uncanny ability to welcome new members into the fold rather quickly. The sense of "we are all in this together" permeates throughout the entire organization. Team members embrace new members to the team and quickly step up to offer assistance and suggestions to ease your transition. Just remember to return the favor when new staff members join your team in the months and years ahead.

Participate in Hobbies

Many nurses new to telephonic care are pleased with their decision to depart from bedside nursing because of the desire to have more time and energy to invest in hobbies and interests. As was previously explained, the amount of energy expended providing care is considerably less. You may find that you have more energy after work to do things that you "always wanted to do" but never had "the time or energy" to do them.

Because of the camaraderie among the staff, you might find or learn of others who share your same interests. Nursing staff have been known to meet together after work to participate in a group activity. This sharing of interests crosses "team" lines and creates a network of friendships and support.

Hours of Work

Probably one of the most stressful aspects of bedside nursing is the lack of control over the work schedule. Hours of work for nursing staff have evolved from the traditional 8-hour day to 10- and 12-hour shifts. Because of shortages, some organizations had to adopt highly flexible scheduling options to attract and maintain nursing staff.

In telephonic environments, the shifts are created to support the clients' needs. Remember, you are calling people who are in their own homes and who might not be living in the same state or time zone as the organization's office. Because of this, shifts rarely start at 7 a.m.

(0700 hours for those who are still on direct care provider thinking mode) and may be of times such as:

- 9 a.m. to 5:30 p.m.
- 10 a.m. to 6:30 p.m.
- Noon to 8:30 p.m.

If an organization is located in the Eastern time zone and clients live on the west coast, shifts might have to span until midnight. Even so, telephonic nurses do not work "night turn." The organization will be aware of any Federal Communication Commission (FCC) laws regarding the times in which clients can be contacted telephonically in the home. Keep in mind, though, that you will not be conducting sales calls, and robocall technology is not used.

Employee Status

The number of hours worked in a pay period is determined by employee status. A full-time employee works the hours identified by the organization in order for the employee to be eligible for all benefits. Some organizations that provide telephonic care hire staff to fill in or work part-time hours. These nurses may hold full-time positions in other organizations and want to earn extra money providing telephonic care.

The hours of work for part-time telephonic nursing staff will also differ. Shifts might be:

- 4 p.m. to 8 p.m.
- 6 p.m. to midnight
- Saturdays only

Extra care and effort must be extended to the nursing staff who are in part-time positions. These nurses do not reap the same personal benefits as other full-time staff and may feel left out or overlooked. Team leaders with part-time staff have to be present and available during these staff members' hours of work to provide assistance and observe care calls. Because it would be unrealistic to expect team leaders to work as much as 16 hours a day, team leaders often schedule their time to cover later shifts and support more than one team.

Care Areas Without Walls

The phrase "hospitals without walls" is commonplace in the health care industry; however, in telephonic care, it is more appropriate to consider the teams and associated clients as being "care areas without walls." Even though you might be assigned to work on one team, there will be times when you will be "pulled" to assist another team to achieve their client care needs and goals. Unlike having to physically leave a direct care area and work with unknown staff and possibly different processes and procedures, you will simply change your dialer selection and provide care to the clients who present to your desktop.

For those nurses who work from a home office, coming into the office regularly helps reinforce and strengthen the teams. It provides time to learn about the other "care areas" in the event the expectation to assist other teams applies to the nurse who works from the home as well.

LONG-TERM SUCCESS

Because telephonic nursing care has been practiced for a few decades, there is no reason to suspect that this approach to client care is going to dissolve any time soon. However, the success of an individual organization will depend on the acceptance of telephonic care as a valid method to improve health and control health care costs.

Telephonic nursing care organizations do not materialize out of thin air. Many people and organizations have invested hours of time and money to establish these businesses. Leadership staff have met for countless hours with health plan, disease management, or wellness program administrators carving out the terms of contracts and expectations. All of this has occurred even before a single position for a staff nurse job was created.

Telephonic care positions are desired by many nurses; however, the job is not for everyone. Organizational human resources departments take great care when interviewing potential staff and make the best possible decisions; however, at times the plan does not work out. New employees may elect to leave a new position immediately at the conclusion of orientation because the position was just not the "right fit." Others have arrived the first day of orientation never to return again. Then there are other staff who might not be "getting it" when providing care and despite frequent counseling and individual training, have to be terminated.

The best advice for any nurse new to telephonic care is to:

- Take care of yourself
- Be responsible for your own learning needs
- Ask questions about anything that you do not understand
- Embrace the philosophy of lifelong learning

A whole new aspect of the health care industry is being opened to you. Enjoy the experience!

KEY POINTS

- Telephonic care expends less energy than direct care.
- Nurses who provide telephonic care may need to alter their lifestyles to maximize personal health.
- Consider adopting approaches suggested to clients to enhance personal wellness such as daily exercise, altering an eating plan, and controlling stress.
- Look forward to making new friends and learning new skills.

Conclusion: The Rest of the Story

This final section has no learning outcomes to achieve, no specific actions to take, or suggestions to overcome challenging care call situations. These final pages serve to summarize the entire text and extend an invitation for you to ask questions for further clarification.

Telephonic care encapsulates many aspects of nursing: communication, therapeutic relationships, assessment, empowerment, legalities, problem solving, clinical decision making, and a few others that I am sure I am forgetting right now. Even so, new skill sets are required and must be developed to be successful in the role of telephonic nurse.

What began as a text to facilitate the telephonic assessment process has evolved into a manual that I hope will support all nurses who desire to take this road in their careers. One of the most frequent questions received when training new telephonic nurses is, "How do I do this job?" I sincerely hope that this question has been answered sufficiently and contributes to your learning.

This last entry in the text is not really a conclusion but a temporary ending. The industry continues to evolve. New processes are being created. New software applications are being developed. And an entirely new crop of telephonic nurses and leadership staff are being prepared to move this aspect of the health care industry into an unknown future.

Examples provided throughout this text were obtained from real situations. Having spent a decade in the industry either providing direct telephonic care or training others to do so, I found it easy to recall the time when a unique situation occurred or a particularly challenging client episode was brought to a successful conclusion. I shared as many of these situations with you as possible.

Although this text might be viewed as a user manual for telephonic nursing care, some things may be missing. But, like any good book, it should leave the reader desiring more. May you desire more and reach out with questions and comments.

When the opportunity to become a telephonic nurse presented itself to me in the late 1990s, I jumped at the chance to "do something different." I had no idea what I was walking into or how my perception of the world of health care would change. It is my hope that you, too, will approach telephonic nursing care with a sense of wonder and high expectations.

Because I embrace and am thankful for receiving feedback, you are encouraged to contact me with any questions, comments, or concerns: dawna.martich@att.net.

Thank you for taking this journey. May you enjoy many more successful years in the profession!

Index

AAACN. *See* American Academy of Ambulatory Care Nursing
ACA. *See* Affordable Care Act
active listening, 13
  assessment techniques, 14–15
  exercises to improve, 21–31
  importance of, 20–21
  telenursing situations with, 33–34
acute hypoglycemia, 297–298
acute illness, 297
Affordable Care Act (ACA), 10
American Academy of Ambulatory Care Nursing (AAACN), 41, 44
American Nursing Credentialing Center (ANCC), 44
American Telemedicine Association
  home telehealth services, 7
  non-face-to-face services, 7
  remote face-to-face services, 6–7
ANCC. *See* American Nursing Credentialing Center
arterial circulation system, 102
  disorders, 213
assessment techniques, for telenursing, 14–15
auscultation, telenursing, 15

blood cells, 102
blood system disorders, 219–221
brain, 153–154

camaraderie, 370
cardiovascular system
  algorithm for, 108–113
  arterial circulation, 102, 213–215
  assessment of, 103
  blood system, 102, 219–221
  disorders, 207, 222
  heart, 101, 208–213
  lymphatic system, 102, 218
  venous circulation, 102, 215–217
care calls, 357–358
cartilage, 137
case management activities, in telephonic care, 357
Centers for Medicare and Medicaid Services (CMS), 5, 6
central nervous system
  brain, 153–154
  spinal cord, 154
change theory, and telephonic nursing care, 318–324
cheat sheets, 361–362
chronic illness, patient/client with, 51–52
clients, issues with, 371–373
clinical documentation, tips to enhance, 352–353
CMS. *See* Centers for Medicare and Medicaid Services
communication, 13
  approaches, sense of hearing, 17–19
  assessment techniques, 14–15
  exercises to improve, 21–31
  telenursing situations with, 32–33
computerized documentation system, 351–353
confidentiality, 54–55
coworkers, 374–376
cranial nerves, 155
credentialing, 44

demographics, 344–345
dental examination, diabetic patients and, 295

diabetes mellitus
    activity and exercise, 294
    acute hypoglycemia, 297–298
    acute illness, 297
    care calls for patients, 299
    clinical manifestations of, 298
    complications of, 290–291
    diagnostic evaluation, 294–295
    disease management program,
        300–301
    medications, 292–293
    nutritional intake, 293
    preventive actions, 295–297
    self-monitoring, 291–292
    types of, 289
diabetic ketoacidosis (DKA), 290
diabetic nerve pain, 296
diagnostic-related groupings (DRGs), 5
diagnostic test, 349
    client adherence to, 340
    importance of, 331
    types of, 331–334
disease management, 373–374
    claims data, 350–351
    patient/client identification, 60–62
DKA. *See* diabetic ketoacidosis
documentation
    avoiding most major mistake
        of all, 353
    information, 343–351
    learning computerized
        documentation system, 351–353
DRGs. *See* diagnostic-related
    groupings

e-mail, 345
exercise/activity, 381–383
    diabetic patients and, 294
experience, in telenursing, 39–41
eye examination, diabetic patients
    and, 295

FDA. *See* Food and Drug
    Administration
female reproductive system, 169

Food and Drug Administration
    (FDA), 348
foot assessment, diabetic patients
    and, 296

gastrointestinal system, 119
    algorithm for, 128–132
    assessment of, 120–121
    primary function of, 119–120
    special situation for, 127
gastrointestinal system, disorders
    of, 225
genitourinary system, 169–182
    disorders, 275

hair follicles, 70
handling stress, 378
hazards of immobility, 380–383
health care professional, 226
Health Information Technology for
    Economic and Clinical Health
    Act (HITECH Act), 57
Health Insurance Portability
    and Accountability Act
    (HIPAA)
    administrative controls/
        enforcement rules, 57
    privacy rules, 56
    security rules, 56–57
health plan, 350–351, 373–374
    information, 349–350
heart, 101
    disorders of, 208–213
hemoglobin A1c blood test, 294
HHS. *See* hyperosmolar
    hyperglycemic state
HIPAA. *See* Health Insurance
    Portability and
    Accountability Act
HITECH Act. *See* Health
    Information Technology
    for Economic and Clinical
    Health Act
HIV/AIDS patients, 303–310
home telehealth services, 7

hyperosmolar hyperglycemic state
(HHS), 290
hypoglycemia, 297–298

ideal work environment, 367, 368
inspection, telenursing, 15
insulin, 292
integumentary system, 69
algorithm for, 82–85
assessment of, 70–78, 85–86
hair follicles, 70
health problems, 78–82
nails, 70
skin, 69–70
integumentary system, disorders
of, 185–190
Internet telephonic care calls, 358
issues/solutions
handling stress, 378
paper, 376–377
people, 371–376
processes, 377

knee-jerk reaction, 375

laboratory tests, 349
client adherence to, 340
importance of, 331
types of, 335–340
layman's terms, 343
lesions, 185–187
Lewin model, 319
licensure, 43–44
lower respiratory tract, 193, 196
lymphatic system, 102
disorders of, 218

mailings, 350
male reproductive system, 170
materials, 350
Medicaid programs, for HIV/AIDS
patients, 304
medications documentation, 347–348

musculoskeletal system, 137
algorithm for, 145–148
assessment of, 138–143, 148
disorders, 243–254
special situations for, 143–145

nails, integumentary system, 70
National Aeronautics and Space
Administration (NASA), 3
National Certification Corporate
(NCC), 44
NCC. *See* National Certification
Corporate
neurological disorders, 259
neurologic system
algorithm for, 162–166
assessment of, 156–162, 166
central nervous system, 153–154
peripheral nervous system, 155–156
noisy patient/client environment, 34
noisy telenursing environment, 33
non-face-to-face services, 7
nurse as client
long-term success, 386–387
personal care, 379–383
stress management, 383–386
nursing process, 313
nursing roles, in telephonic care,
356–358

open communication, 327–328
oral agents, for diabetes mellitus,
292–293

palpation, telenursing, 15
patient care, and telenursing, 10–11
patient/client identification, 47–49
barriers, 49
chronic illness, 51–52
confidentiality, 54–55
disease management, 60
Health Information Technology
for Economic and Clinical
Health Act, 57

patient/client identification (*cont.*)
Health Insurance Portability and
Accountability Act, 55–57
posthospitalization, 57
wellness program, 52–54, 63
patient/client personal
information, 32
percussion, telenursing, 15
peripheral nervous system
cranial nerves, 155
spinal nerves, 156
personal care, 379–383
personal/protected health
information (PHI), 56
PHI. *See* personal/protected health
information
physical activity, diabetic patients
and, 294
physical assessment data, 347
posthospital care, 356–357
primary lesions, 185, 186

rashes, skin disorders, 187–188
recognize health problems, 382–383
reminder calls, 358
remote face-to-face services, 6–7
resources, telephonic care, 355–356
respiratory system, 89
assessment of, 90, 91
disorders of, 193
lower, 193, 196
upper, 193, 194
by listening, 94

saving input information, 353
secondary lesions, 185, 186–187
self-monitoring, 291–292
sense of hearing, 17–21
senses
used in patient/client care, 13–14
used in telenursing, 16–17
sensory system, 156
algorithm for, 162–166
assessment of, 156–157, 166
sensory system, disorders of,
259–260, 267–269

skin
integumentary system, 69–70
skin disorders
lesions, 185–187
rashes, 187–189
trauma, 189–190
smoking
and diabetes mellitus, 297
spinal cord, 154
spinal nerves, 156
standards of clinical practice, 41–42
standards of professional
performance, 42
static resources, 376–377
stress management, 383–386

telemedicine, reimbursement for, 7–8
telenursing, 3
active listening in, 33–34
American Telemedicine
Association, 6–7
with communication, 32–33
credentialing, 44
current reimbursement for, 7–8
health care industry changes, 10
history of, 3–4
impact on medical practice, 4–5
licensure, 43–44
patient care through, 10–11
reimbursement issues, 5–6
senses used in, 16–17
standards of clinical practice,
41–42
standards of professional
performance, 42
telehealth and telemedicine, 9–10
telephone system, 364
"telephonic 20," 379
telephonic nursing care
change theory, application of,
320–324
cheat sheets, 361–362
information and support, 316–317
nursing process, 313
open communication, 327–328
other resources, 358–360
positions, 386

practice patterns, 360–361
resources, 355–356
roles for, 356–358
teaching, 314–318, 324–327
work environments. *See* work
environments
transtheoretical model of change,
319–320
type 1 diabetes mellitus, 289
type 2 diabetes mellitus, 289

upper respiratory tract, 193, 194

venous circulation system, 102
disorders of, 215

weight management, 379–380
diabetes mellitus, 293
welcome calls, 357
wellness program, 373–374
patient/client enrolled in, 52–54,
63–64
wellness program information,
349–350
windows-based operating system, 343
work environments
call center, 363–365
home, 366–367
ideal, 367
work issues, 368–370

Zidovudine (AZT), 307

Printed in the United States
By Bookmasters